# BEDSIDE

# ULTRASOUND

## LEVEL 1

## PETER STEINMETZ MD

### SECOND EDITION

Includes online instructional videos at:
bedsideultrasoundlevel1.com

Also available as an iBook with embedded videos.

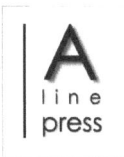

A
line
press

Bedside Ultrasound – Level 1    ISBN: 978-0-9919566-8-5

*First Edition*
   *first printing, June 2013*
   *second printing, October 2013*
   *third printing, February 2014; revisions include new figures (Figures 3.6, 7.6, 10.2), new figures in the 'Case closed' section of each chapter, expanded Summary (page 78), and correction of minor typographical errors.*
*Second Edition*
   *first printing, August 2018; this second edition includes improved and updated chapters, and the Canadian Point of Care Ultrasound Society guidelines. We also added false-positives and false-negatives for each of the indications. Overall, this book includes new text (44 pages), new illustrations to better illustrate important concepts (29 figures), and new instructional videos (2 videos).*

The information in this book is designed to provide helpful information on the subjects discussed. While best efforts have been made to provide accurate information that is in accord with current standards of practice, the author, editor, or publisher make no warranty with respect to the accuracy or completeness of the contents. Application of the information in a particular situation remains the professional responsibility of the physician. Any likeness to actual persons in the case studies is strictly coincidental. References are provided for informational purposes only and do not constitute endorsement of websites or other sources.

**Scientific editor**
Sharon Oleskevich PhD

**Web manager for online videos**
John D. Clements PhD

**Proofreader**
Christiane de Brentani BA

**Printer**
IngramSpark / Lightning Source Inc.

**Publisher**
A-line Press, Montreal, Canada

# PREFACE

This introductory handbook is a practical reference for healthcare workers starting to apply bedside ultrasound in their daily practice. It aims to articulate the practical and cognitive skills necessary to effectively use this tool.

In this second edition, we have improved and updated each chapter, and added the Canadian Point of Care Ultrasound Society guidelines. We also added false-positives and false-negatives for each of the indications. Overall, this book includes new text (44 pages), new illustrations to better illustrate important concepts (29 figures), and new instructional videos (2 videos).

The instructional ultrasound videos can be accessed at:

**bedsideultrasoundlevel1.com**

# DEDICATION

*"My only question is, why haven't we done this sooner?"*

*Arnold Steinberg, 2012*

This textbook is dedicated to the late Arnold Steinberg whose vision and support were instrumental in establishing the bedside ultrasound curriculum at McGill University.

# ABOUT THE AUTHOR

Dr. Peter Steinmetz is an Assistant Professor in the Department of Family Medicine at McGill University. He founded and leads undergraduate bedside ultrasound teaching at McGill University. As an executive board member of the Canadian Point of Care Ultrasound Society, he helps set national certification standards for ultrasound use in the family physician's office. He has published on the accuracy and skill acquisition of medical students using bedside ultrasound. He has also been invited to teach bedside ultrasound in Asia (Thailand) and Africa (Rwanda) and co-directed the World Congress of Ultrasound in Medical Education.

Dr. Steinmetz currently works at a community health clinic where point of care ultrasound is actively used in a family medicine setting.

# ACKNOWLEDGEMENTS

There are countless people who deserve mention and a word of thanks for inspiring this second edition. They include the hundreds of McGill medical students who used this book to learn ultrasound and gave constructive feedback over the last five years of our groundbreaking bedside ultrasound curriculum. I am also thankful to the Canadian Point of Care Ultrasound Society for providing clear guidelines for bedside ultrasound use by Canadian clinicians as outlined at the end of relevant chapters. For the French edition, I am grateful to Dr. Claude Topping for his precise translations as well as important additions to the text itself.

A special thanks to Sharon Oleskevich for countless hours of editing, design, organization, writing, and general good advice.

*P.S.*

# CONTENTS

## 1. ULTRASOUND BASICS                                               1

  1.1  What is ultrasound?                                     1
  1.2  How do ultrasound probes send and receive ultrasound?  3
  1.3  How does ultrasound behave travelling through tissue?  4
       Attenuation                                          4
       Reflection                                           5
  1.4  Gain                                                    7
  1.5  Depth                                                   8
  1.6  Resolution and penetration                             10
  1.7  Doppler and flow                                       12

## 2. IMAGE GENERATION                                               15

  2.1  Probe choice                                           15
  2.2  Sonographer and patient position                       17
  2.3  Use of gel                                             19
  2.4  Identification of structures                           20
  2.5  Orientation of image                                   22
       Imaging planes                                       22
       Field of view                                        24
       Orientation of structures relative to probe position  26
  2.6  Adjustment of depth                                    28
  2.7  Adjustment of gain                                     29
  2.8  Cleaning machine and probe between patients            29
  2.9  Troubleshooting tips                                   30

## 3. IMAGE ARTIFACTS                                               31

| | | |
|---|---|---|
| 3.1 | Common artifacts | 31 |
| 3.2 | Shadowing artifact | 32 |
| | Advantage | 32 |
| | Disadvantage | 33 |
| 3.3 | Enhancement artifact | 34 |
| | Advantage | 34 |
| | Disadvantage | 35 |
| 3.4 | Mirror image artifact | 36 |
| | Advantage | 36 |
| | Disadvantage | 36 |
| 3.5 | Reverberation artifact | 37 |
| | Advantage | 37 |
| 3.6 | Refraction (edge) artifact | 38 |
| 3.7 | Troubleshooting tips | 39 |

## 4. DYSPNEA                                                       41

| | | |
|---|---|---|
| 4.1 | Probe choice | 43 |
| 4.2 | Patient position and scanning technique - Anterior chest exam | 44 |
| 4.3 | Lung sliding | 45 |
| | Clinical relevance - Pneumothorax | 45 |
| 4.4 | 'A' lines | 50 |
| 4.5 | 'B' lines | 51 |
| 4.6 | Lung profiles | 52 |
| | Clinical relevance - 'A' profile | 52 |
| | Clinical relevance - 'B' profile | 52 |
| | Clinical relevance - 'AB' profile | 52 |
| 4.7 | Posterolateral chest exam | 54 |
| | Clinical relevance - Pleural effusion and lung consolidation | 55 |
| 4.8 | Troubleshooting tips | 58 |
| 4.9 | False-positives and false-negatives | 59 |
| 4.10 | CPoCUS documentation standards | 59 |

## 5. Undifferentiated hypotension    61

5.1  Probe choice                                                63
5.2  Patient position and scanning technique                     63
5.3  Left ventricular function                                   64
    Clinical relevance - LV dysfunction                      69
5.4  Right to left ventricular diameter ratio                    70
    Clinical relevance - Pulmonary embolism                  70
5.5  Pericardial effusion                                        71
    Clinical relevance - Cardiac tamponade                   72
5.6  Volume status and the IVC                                   73
    Clinical relevance - Hypotensive patient                 76
5.7  Additional ultrasound assessments for hypotension           78
5.8  Troubleshooting tips                                        79
5.9  False-positives and false-negatives                         80
5.10 CPoCUS documentation standards                              81

## 6. Trauma    83

6.1  Probe choice                                                85
6.2  Patient position and scanning technique                     85
6.3  The eFAST algorithm                                         86
    Question #1: Does the patient have a hemoperitoneum?     87
    Question #2: Does the patient have a hemopericardium?    95
    Question #3: Does the patient have a hemothorax?         96
    Question #4: Does the patient have a pneumothorax?       97
6.4  Troubleshooting tips                                        98
6.5  False-positives and false-negatives                         98
6.6  CPoCUS documentation standards                              100

## 7. Abdominal aortic aneurysm (AAA)    103

7.1  Probe choice                                                105
7.2  Patient position and scanning technique                     106
7.3  Using bedside ultrasound to identify an AAA                 110
    Clinical relevance - Abdominal aortic aneurysm           110
7.4  Troubleshooting tips                                        113
7.5  False-positives and false-negatives                         114
7.6  CPoCUS documentation standards                              114

## 8. CHOLECYSTITIS                                                        117

8.1   Probe choice                                                     119
8.2   Patient position and scanning technique                         120
      Scanning technique #1: The subcostal sweep                      120
      Scanning technique #2: Left lateral decubitus                   121
      Scanning technique #3: The X-7 approach                         121
      Scanning technique #4: The posterolateral approach              122
8.3   Ultrasound appearance of the gallbladder                        123
      Clinical relevance - Cholecystitis                              126
8.4   Troubleshooting tips                                            134
8.5   False-positives and false-negatives                            135
8.6   CPoCUS documentation standards                                  135

## 9. KIDNEY INJURY                                                        137

9.1   Probe choice                                                     139
9.2   Patient position and scanning technique                         140
      Imaging the kidney in the coronal plane                         140
      Imaging the bladder in the sagittal plane                       143
      Imaging the bladder in the transverse plane                     144
9.3   Obstructive causes of kidney injury                             145
      Clinical relevance - Hydronephrosis                             145
      Clinical relevance - Post-void bladder volume                   147
      Clinical relevance - Acute vs. chronic kidney injury            149
      Clinical relevance - Other pathology                            150
9.4   Troubleshooting tips                                            152
9.5   CPoCUS documentation standards                                  153

## 10. DEEP VENOUS THROMBOSIS (DVT)
   OF THE LOWER LIMB                                                   155

10.1 Probe choice                                                     157
10.2 Patient position and scanning technique -
     Common femoral vein                                              158
      Clinical relevance - DVT in the common femoral vein             158
10.3 Patient position and scanning technique -
     Popliteal vein                                                   164
      Clinical relevance - DVT in the popliteal vein                  165

10.4  Troubleshooting tips                                      166
10.5  False-positives and false-negatives                       167
10.6  CPoCUS documentation standards                            168

## 11. ECTOPIC PREGNANCY                                        171

11.1  Probe choice                                              173
11.2  Patient position and scanning technique                   174
    Imaging the uterus in the sagittal plane                    174
    Imaging the uterus in the transverse plane                  175
11.3  Criteria for diagnosing an intra-uterine pregnancy (IUP)  176
    Clinical relevance - Ectopic pregnancy                      180
    Clinical relevance - Other pathology                        180
11.4  Troubleshooting tips                                      181
11.5  False-positives and false-negatives                       182
11.6  CPoCUS documentation standards                            183

## INDEX                                                        185
## REFERENCES                                                   189

# 1. ULTRASOUND BASICS

1.1  What is ultrasound?

1.2  How do ultrasound probes send and receive ultrasound?

1.3  How does ultrasound behave travelling through tissue?

1.4  Gain

1.5  Depth

1.6  Resolution and penetration

1.7  Doppler and flow

## 1.1 What is ultrasound?

Ultrasound is a sound wave that oscillates with a frequency greater than 20,000 Hz (20,000 cycles per second or 20 kHz). The human ear can detect sound waves with frequencies between 0.02-20 kHz. Sound waves above 20 kHz, such as those generated by dog whistles, bat calls, and ultrasound machines, cannot be interpreted as sound by the human ear. These high frequency sound waves are called **ultrasound**.

It is useful to understand some basic concepts about ultrasound in order to correctly interpret the images generated by the bedside ultrasound machine.

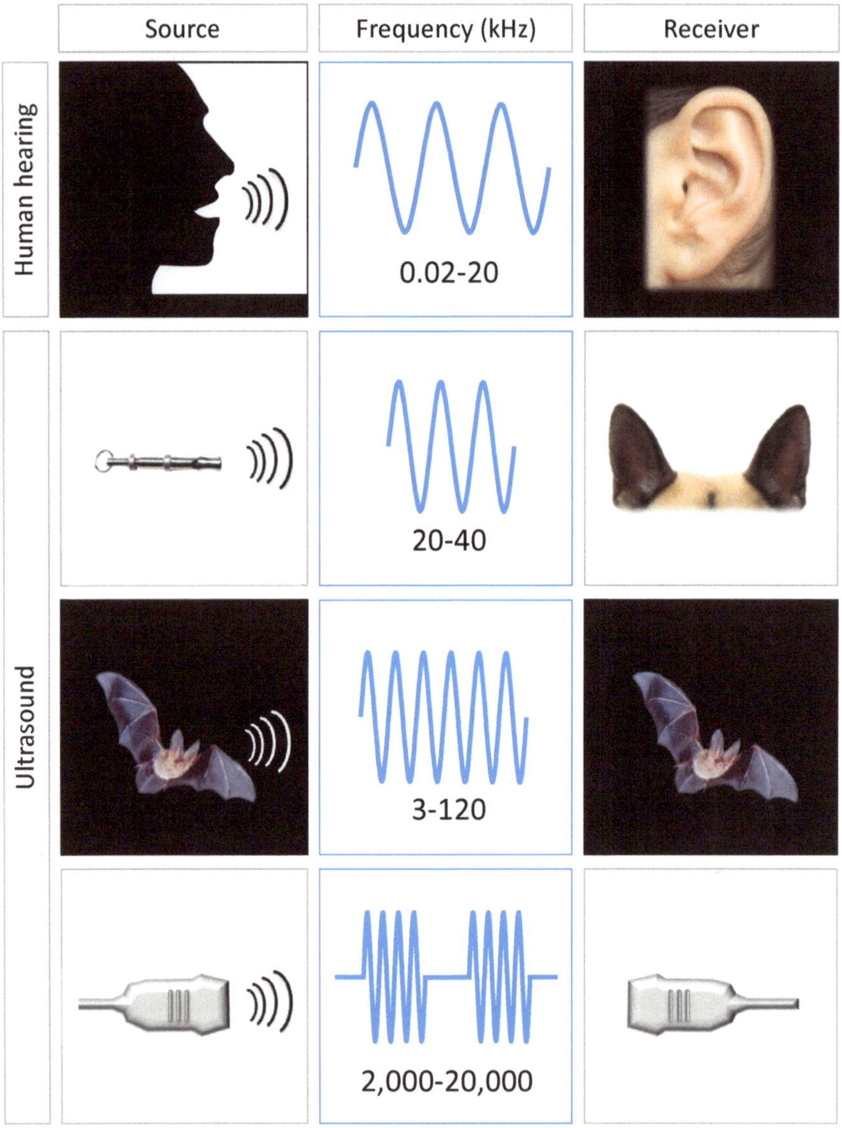

| Source | Frequency (kHz) | Receiver |
|---|---|---|
| Human hearing | 0.02-20 | |
| Ultrasound | 20-40 | |
| | 3-120 | |
| | 2,000-20,000 | |

**Figure 1.1 Different sound wave frequencies.**
The human ear can interpret sound waves with frequencies up to 20 kHz. Sound waves with frequencies above 20 kHz are termed ultrasound. Ultrasound probes emit frequencies from 2,000-20,000 kHz (2-20 MHz).

## 1.2 How do ultrasound probes send and receive ultrasound?

Ultrasound probes have two functions: to send and receive ultrasound. An ultrasound probe spends 1% of its time sending sound waves and 99% of its time receiving sound waves.

The probe starts by sending out bursts of ultrasound. When ultrasound encounters a structure, it reflects off that structure and returns to the probe. The reflected ultrasound is interpreted and expressed as an image on the ultrasound machine monitor.

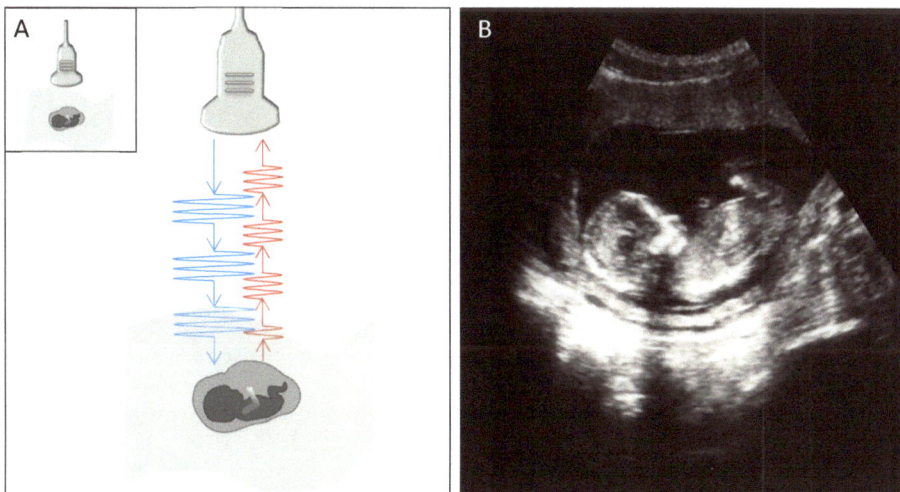

**Figure 1.2 Ultrasound probes send and receive ultrasound.**
**A.** Schematic demonstrating a probe sending sound waves (blue) and receiving the reflected returning sound waves (red).
**B.** The returning sound waves are detected by the probe and translated into an ultrasound image.

## 1.3 How does ultrasound behave travelling through tissue?

**Attenuation**

Attenuation describes the dampening of the amplitude of ultrasound as it travels through tissue. Attenuation occurs as ultrasound energy is converted into heat, absorbed by a structure, reflected back to the probe, or scattered away from the probe.

Attenuation is directly proportional to the distance that the ultrasound travels and to the ultrasound frequency. Attenuation is also affected by the characteristics of the medium encountered.

**Distance:** Attenuation of ultrasound increases as the ultrasound propagates deeper into the body. When imaging the abdomen, the far-field (deeper) structures can appear darker due to attenuation of the ultrasound.

**Frequency:** High frequency ultrasound attenuates more rapidly than low frequency ultrasound. Thus, high frequency probes cannot be used to image deep structures.

**Type of medium:** Air and bone cause a high degree of attenuation. Fluid causes a low degree of attenuation.

## Reflection

An image is generated by the ultrasound waves that are reflected from a structure and returned to the probe. The image appears brighter as the amount of reflection increases. In general, reflection is greatest when ultrasound encounters a structure of high-density or when it crosses an interface between structures of different densities.

**Hyperechoic:** Bone appears hyperechoic (**white**) on the ultrasound image. Its high-density and the interface between surrounding structures of lower density cause a high degree of reflection.

**Hypoechoic:** Muscle and liver appear hypoechoic (**grey**) on the ultrasound image due to their moderate density.

**Anechoic:** Fluid (blood, ascites, pleural effusions) appears anechoic (**black**) on the ultrasound image. This is because ultrasound travels through low-density structures with minimal attenuation and reflection back to the ultrasound probe.

**Table 1.1 Ultrasound image terminology**

| Terminology | Appearance on ultrasound image | Medium | Density of structure |
|---|---|---|---|
| Hyperechoic | White | Bone | High |
| Hypoechoic | Grey | Muscle, liver | Moderate |
| Anechoic | Black | Fluid | Low |

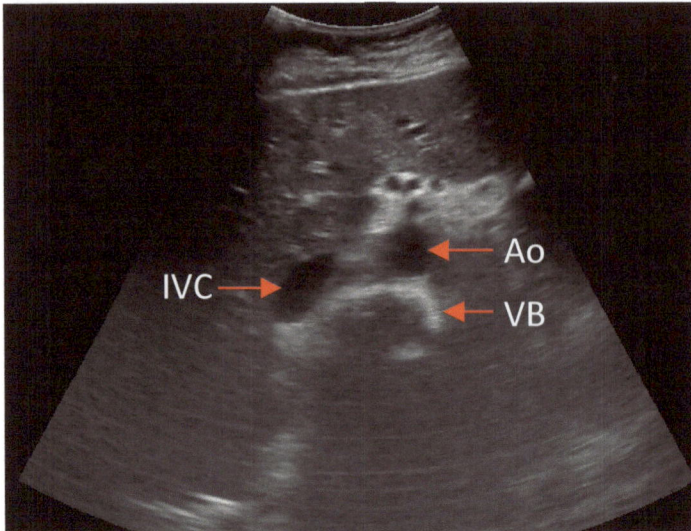

**Figure 1.3 Appearance of structures with different densities.**
The vertebral body (VB) is a bony, high-density structure that appears hyperechoic (white) on the ultrasound image. The aorta (Ao) and inferior vena cava (IVC) are low-density structures that appear anechoic (black). The tissues surrounding these structures are of moderate density and so appear hypoechoic (varying shades of grey).

## 1.4 Gain

Due to the attenuation of the ultrasound returning to the probe, structures may appear dark and hard to identify on the image. Increasing the gain on the ultrasound machine increases the amplification of the reflected ultrasound. This adjustment makes structures appear hyperechoic (white) on the screen and easier to identify.

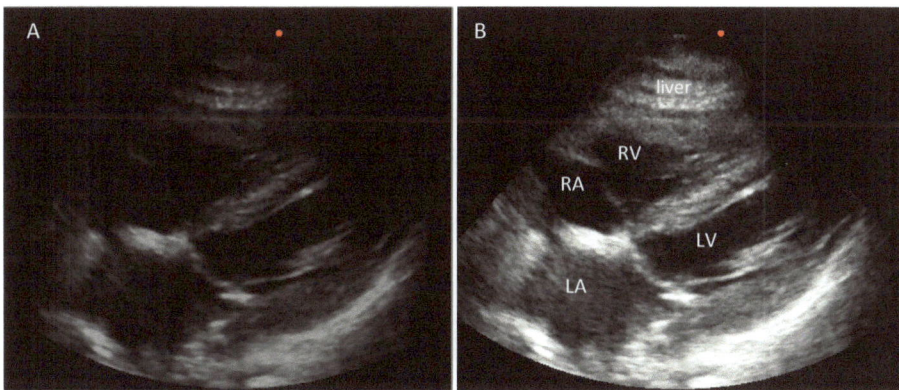

**Figure 1.4 Gain adjustment.**
**A.** Ultrasound image showing a subxiphoid view of the heart. With low gain, structures appear dark on the screen.
**B.** Same image with high gain, structures now appear brighter on the screen.
LV: left ventricle, LA: left atrium, RA: right atrium, RV: right ventricle.

## 1.5 Depth

Ultrasound machines estimate the depth of a structure by measuring the time it takes for a waveform to leave the probe, reflect off a structure, and return to the probe.

Ultrasound striking superficial structures will return to the probe first, followed by ultrasound returning after striking deeper structures. For example, if you are performing an ultrasound of the abdomen on a supine patient, the aorta lies superficial to the vertebral bodies. Therefore, an ultrasound waveform leaving the probe will reflect off the aorta and return to the probe before it reflects off the vertebral body and returns to the probe. The ultrasound machine interprets this time difference and generates an image with the aorta superficial to the vertebral body.

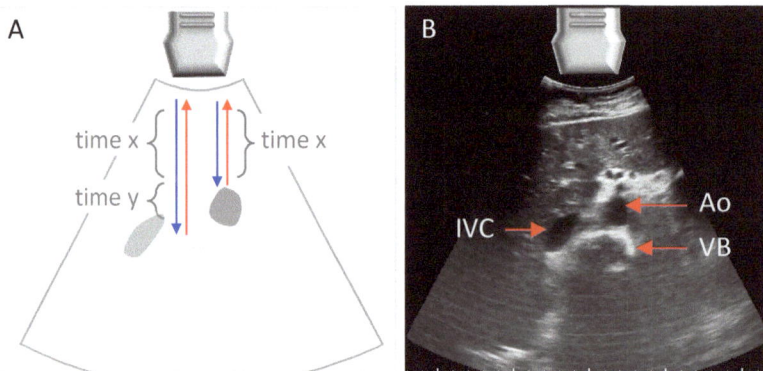

**Figure 1.5 Ultrasound machines estimate the depth of a structure.**
**A.** The depth of the structure determines the time for ultrasound to travel from the probe to the structure (blue arrow) and back again (red arrow). The round-trip time is longer for deeper structures (time x + time y) compared to more superficial structures (time x).
**B.** Corresponding ultrasound image demonstrating the aorta (Ao) superficial to the vertebral body (VB). IVC: inferior vena cava.

The depth of the ultrasound field can be adjusted by changing how often the signal is emitted from the probe. Adjust the depth setting on the ultrasound machine such that structures of interest can be viewed in the middle of the ultrasound field.

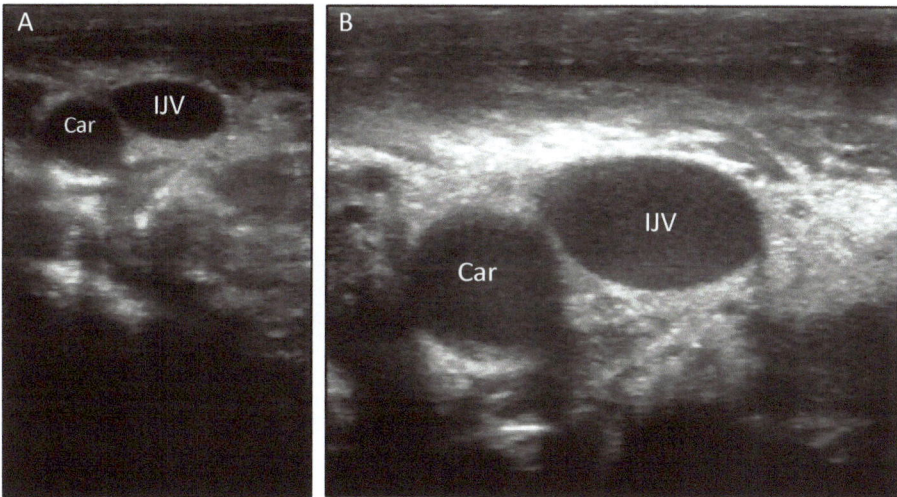

**Figure 1.6 Depth adjustment.**
**A.** Depth setting is too high. The internal jugular vein (IJV) is too high in the field of view and difficult to identify.
**B.** Lower depth setting. Same vessels in the middle of the field appear larger and easier to identify. Car: carotid artery.

## 1.6 Resolution and penetration

The frequency of the ultrasound affects image resolution and tissue penetration in the following two ways:

**Principle #1:**   The frequency of the ultrasound is proportional to the degree of resolution:

- Low frequency sound waves provide low resolution

- High frequency sound waves provide high resolution.

**Principle #2:**   The frequency of the ultrasound is inversely proportional to the degree of penetration:

- Low frequency sound waves penetrate a greater distance and are used to image deep structures

- High frequency sound waves penetrate a shorter distance and are used to image superficial structures.

**Practical application:**

A low frequency ultrasound probe is a good choice to produce low resolution images of deep structures.

A high frequency ultrasound probe is a good choice to produce high resolution images of superficial structures.

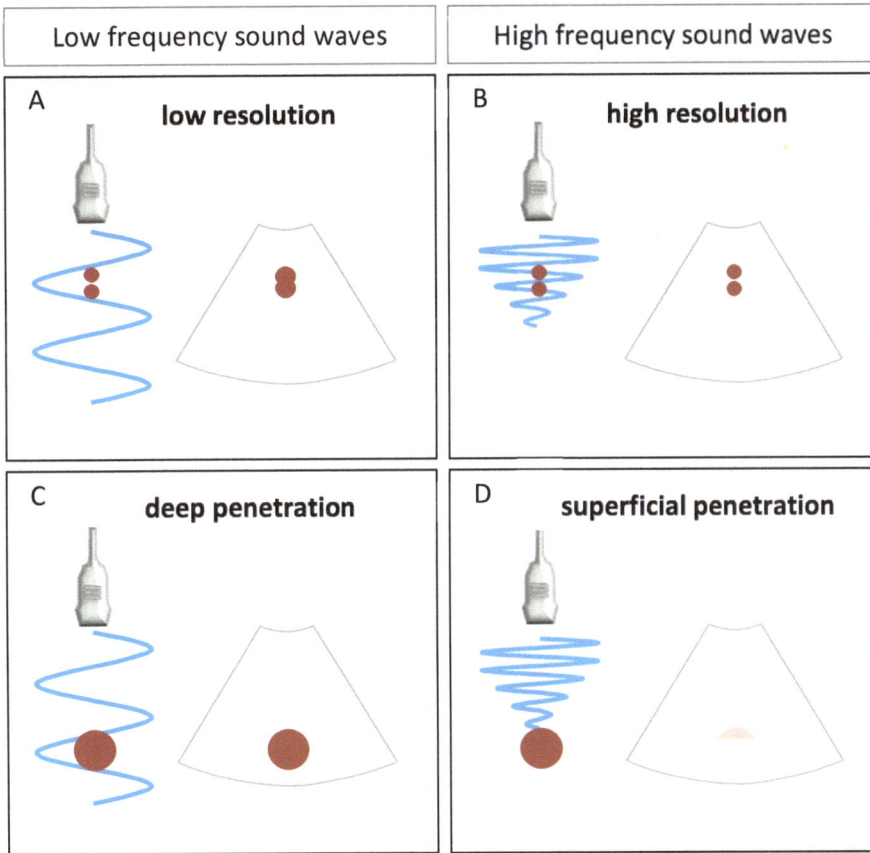

**Figure 1.7 Frequency of ultrasound dictates resolution and penetration.**
**A.** Low frequency sound waves provide a low resolution ultrasound image.
**B.** High frequency sound waves provide a high resolution ultrasound image.
**C.** Low frequency sound waves can image deep structures.
**D.** High frequency sound waves cannot image deep structures.

## 1.7 Doppler and flow

As ultrasound is reflected from moving objects like flowing blood, the frequency of the returning waveform is altered. This frequency shift is described by the Doppler principle. The frequency of the reflected ultrasound is increased when blood flow is towards the probe. The frequency of the reflected ultrasound is decreased when blood flow is away from the probe.

The direction of blood flow relative to the probe is represented by different colors on the ultrasound image. One commonly used convention is that flow away from the probe is colored blue and flow towards the probe is colored red. This convention can be remembered using the acronym **BART**.

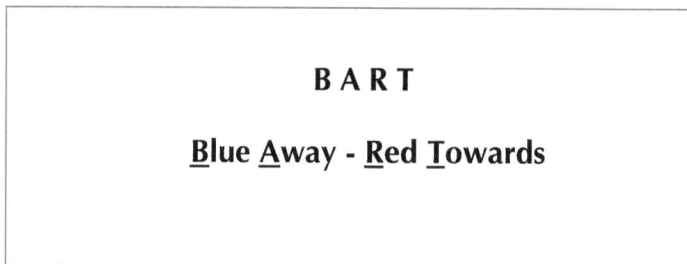

**B A R T**

**Blue Away - Red Towards**

The Doppler principle is useful for differentiating arteries from veins. As shown in Figure 1.8, when the ultrasound beam is directed caudally and towards the heart (A-B), flow in the jugular vein is away from the probe (blue) and flow in the carotid artery is towards the probe (red).

Reversing the ultrasound beam by pointing the probe cephalad (C-D) reverses the colored representations because the direction of flow relative to the probe has been reversed.

There is no frequency shift when the ultrasound beam is directed perpendicular to blood flow (E-F) and therefore there is no colored representation.

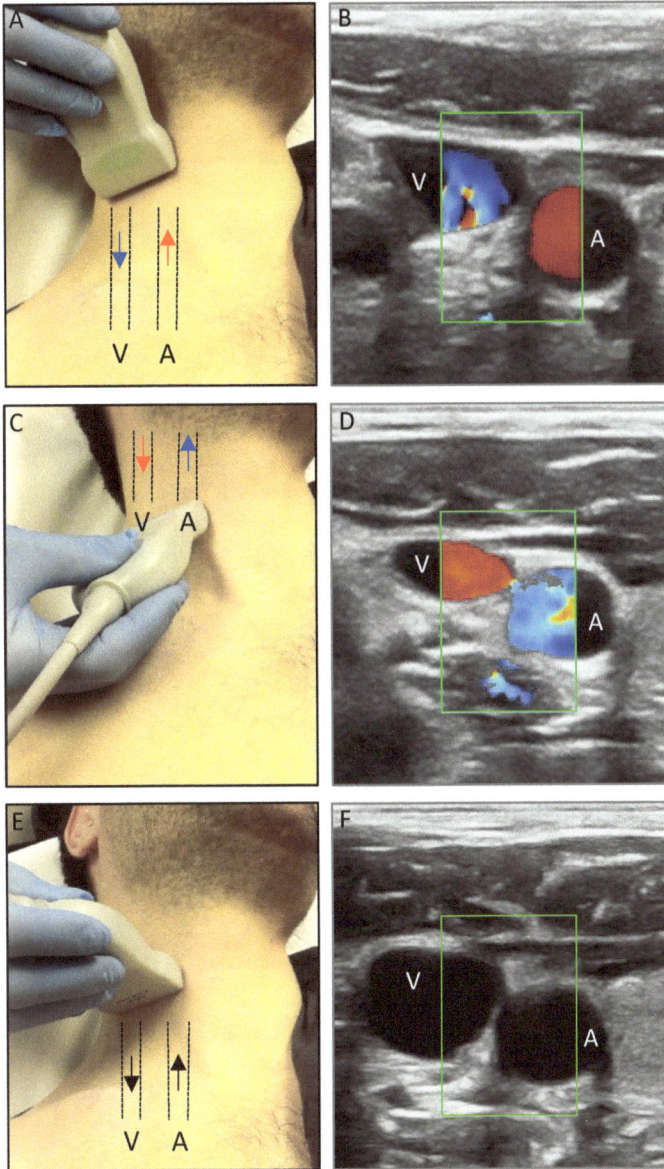

**Figure 1.8 Using Doppler and 'BART' to assess direction of blood flow.**
**A-B.** When the probe is pointing caudally, venous flow is away from the probe (blue) and arterial flow is towards the probe (red).
**C-D.** When the probe is pointing cephalad, venous flow is towards the probe (red) and arterial flow is away from the probe (blue).
**E-F.** No color is generated when the probe is held perpendicular to flow.
V: Jugular vein, A: Carotid artery.

# 2. IMAGE GENERATION

2.1  Probe choice

2.2  Sonographer and patient position

2.3  Use of gel

2.4  Identification of structures

2.5  Orientation of image

2.6  Adjustment of depth

2.7  Adjustment of gain

2.8  Cleaning machine and probe between patients

2.9  Troubleshooting tips

## 2.1 Probe choice

The choice of probe depends on the depth of the structure being imaged. Low frequency probes provide the penetration necessary to image deep structures. High frequency probes provide excellent imaging of small superficial structures.

## Table 2.1 Appropriate probe choice for imaging different structures

| Low frequency probe (2-6 MHz) | High frequency probe (5-14 MHz) |
|---|---|
| Heart | Vessels |
| Gallbladder | Nerves |
| Kidney | Pleura |
| Bladder | Eye |
| Liver | Soft tissue |
| Spleen | Testicle |

| Low frequency phased array probe | Low frequency curvilinear probe | High frequency linear probe |
|---|---|---|
| A | B | C |

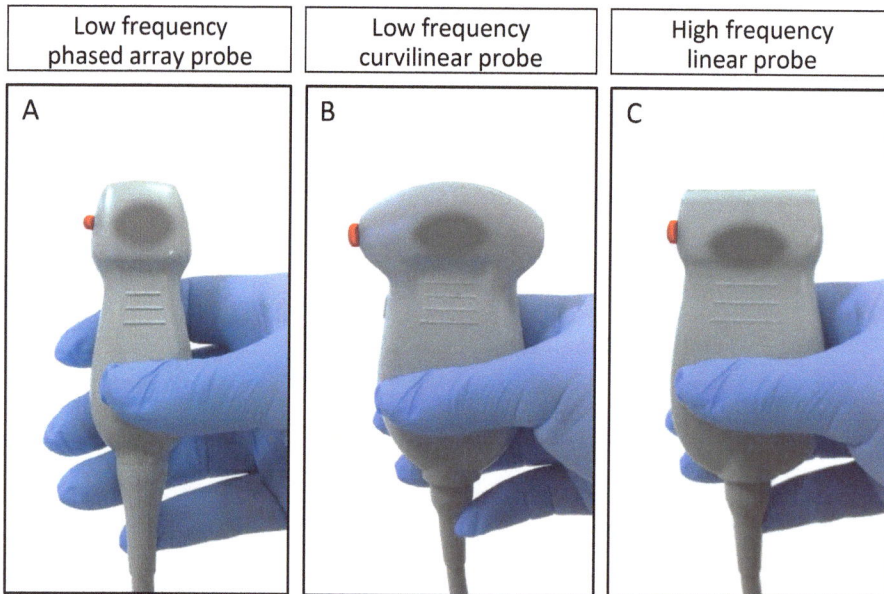

## Figure 2.1 Three commonly used probes.
**A.** The low frequency phased array probe is used for imaging heart, lung, and abdomen.
**B.** The low frequency curvilinear probe is used for imaging abdominal structures.
**C.** The high frequency linear probe is used for imaging superficial structures. Red circle denotes orientation marker.

## 2.2 Sonographer and patient position

The position of both the sonographer and the patient must be optimized to ensure acquisition of high quality images. The height of the patient's bed should be adjusted so that the ultrasonographer is comfortable. Awkward positioning will cause the ultrasonographer to tire and be unable to obtain adequate images. Resting part of the hand on the patient may decrease fatigue, enhance image stability, and enable small, controlled movements.

Due to space and time constraints in bedside ultrasound, the sonographer should learn to obtain images from either side of the patient.

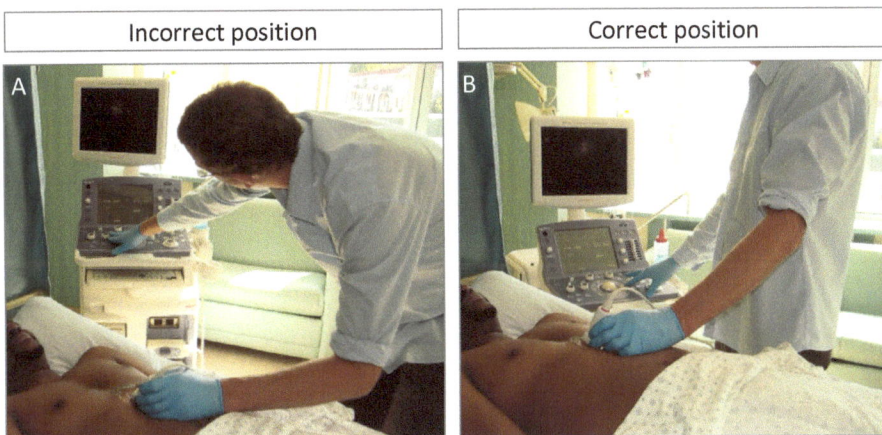

**Figure 2.2 Ultrasonographer position.**
**A. Incorrect position:** the bed is too low and the screen is facing away from the sonographer. The ultrasonographer will soon tire and is unlikely to generate adequate images.
**B. Correct position:** the ultrasonographer is well placed to orient the probe, view the screen, and adjust settings.

There are many examples when the patient's position is important to obtain optimal images.

### Table 2.2 Patient position for optimal ultrasound images

| Area of interest | Patient position for optimal images |
| --- | --- |
| Lung | Supine or semi-seated depending on indication |
| Heart - subxiphoid view | Supine |
| Kidney - left | Supine or right lateral decubitus |
| Kidney - right | Supine or left lateral decubitus |
| Gallbladder | Supine or left lateral decubitus |
| Free abdominal / intraperitoneal fluid | Supine |
| Aorta | Supine |
| Neck veins | Supine |
| Leg veins for deep venous thrombosis (DVT) | Supine with head elevated, or sitting for ambulatory patients |

## 2.3 Use of gel

Ultrasound waves scatter when they encounter air and this greatly diminishes the reflected ultrasound signal. To avoid air being trapped between the probe surface and the patient's body, gel is applied between the probe surface and the body. The gel allows the ultrasound waves to travel between the probe and the body without scattering.

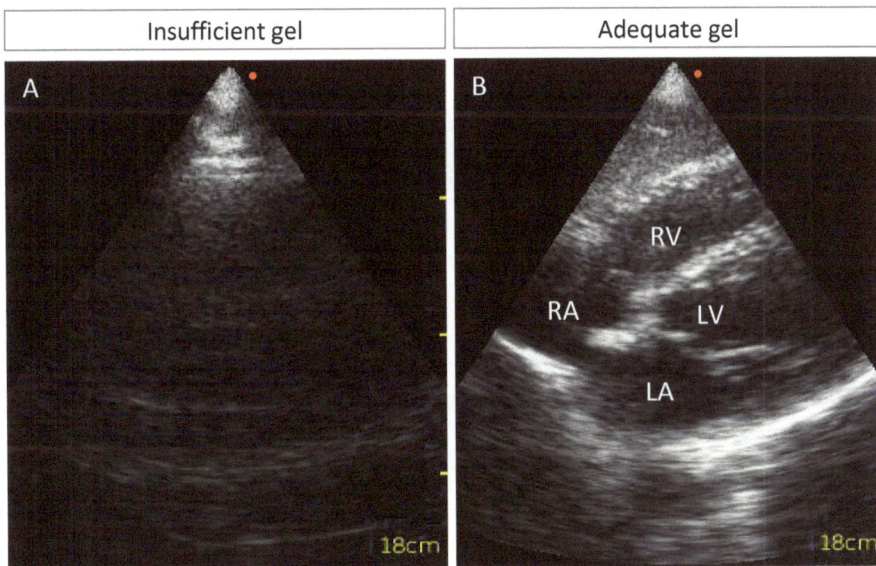

**Figure 2.3 Two subxiphoid images of the heart.**
**A.** The image to the left was obtained with insufficient gel, resulting in an artifact obscuring the heart.
**B.** Same view but with adequate gel applied.
LV: left ventricle, LA: left atrium, RA: right atrium, RV: right ventricle. Red circle denotes orientation marker.

## 2.4 Identification of structures

As the probe contacts the patient, slowly scan until the structure of interest appears on the monitor of the ultrasound machine. Adjustments to the probe position are required to center the structure of interest on the ultrasound image.

Probes can either be rotated, tilted (to sweep through the structure), or rocked. Once in position, the examiner can also slide the probe in the antero-posterior or infero-superior direction.

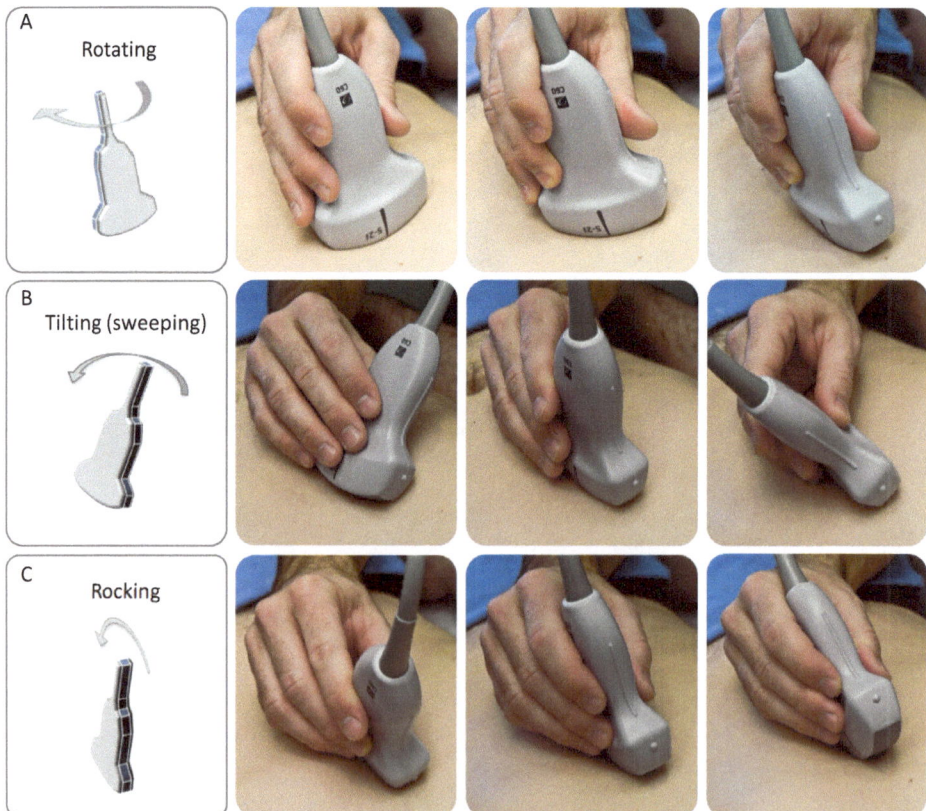

**Figure 2.4 Common terminology for probe movements.**
Modified with permission from [1].

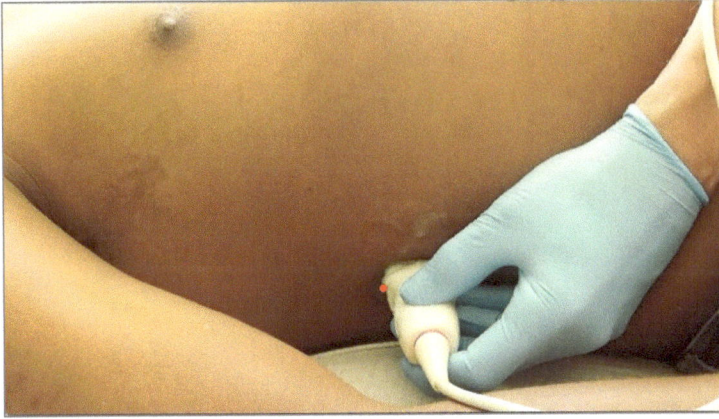

**Video 2.1 Scan slowly to identify the structure of interest.**
The probe must be moved slowly to identify the right kidney. Red circle denotes
orientation marker. Video: bedsideultrasoundlevel1.com

## 2.5 Orientation of image

**Imaging planes**

The body is divided into sagittal, coronal, and transverse planes.

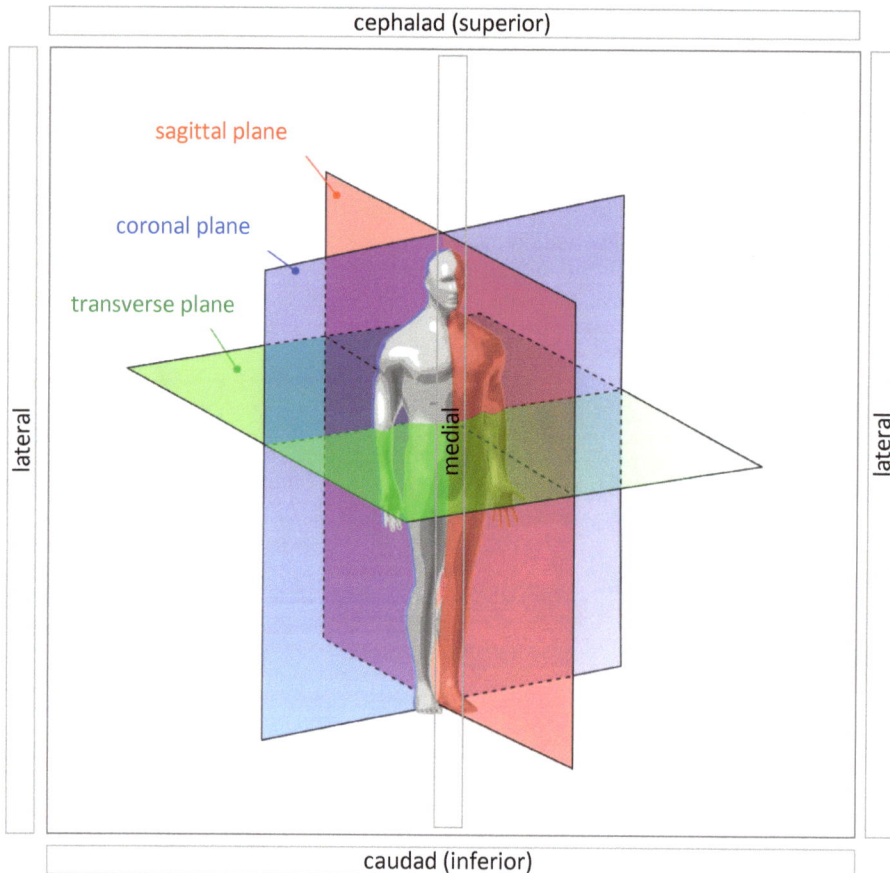

cephalad (superior)

sagittal plane

coronal plane

transverse plane

lateral

medial

lateral

caudad (inferior)

**Figure 2.5 Body planes and orientation [2].**

As the structure of interest appears on the ultrasound machine monitor, the plane of the image is dictated by the orientation of the ultrasound probe.

For example, to obtain an image of the abdomen in the sagittal plane, the probe is placed on the anterior abdomen with the orientation marker pointing cephalad.

To obtain an image of the abdomen in the coronal plane, the probe is placed over the lateral abdomen with the orientation marker pointing cephalad.

To obtain an image of the abdomen in the transverse plane, the probe is placed on the anterior abdomen with the orientation marker pointing to the patient's right.

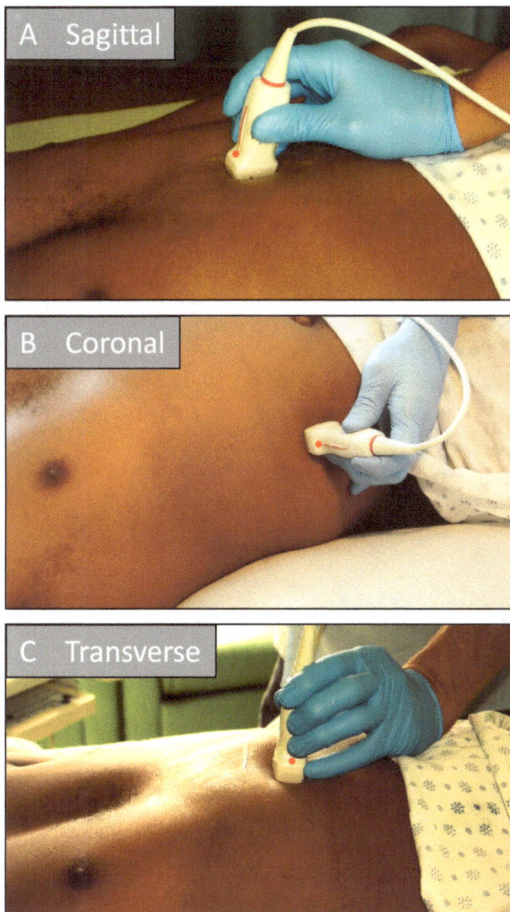

**Figure 2.6 Probe placement.**
Probe placement for generation of abdominal images in the sagittal (A), coronal (B), and transverse (C) planes. Red circle denotes orientation marker.

## Field of view

Ultrasound probes generate different shaped fields of view on the ultrasound monitor. For example, low frequency phased array or curvilinear probes generate triangular fields of view. High frequency linear probes generate rectangular fields of view.

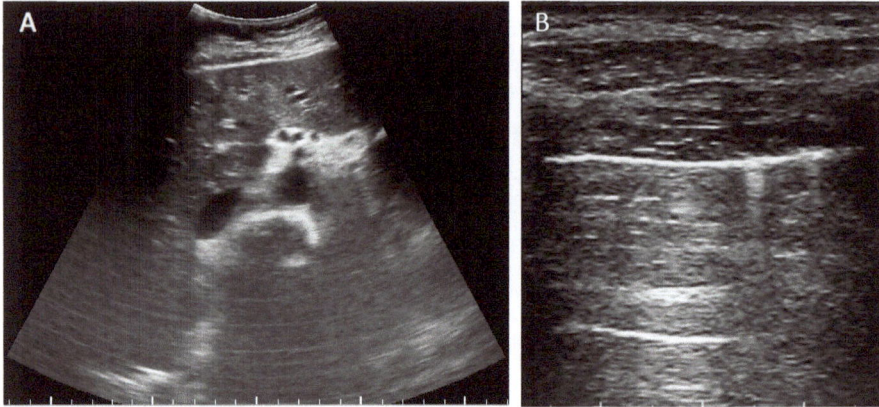

**Figure 2.7 Fields of view generated by different probes.**
**A.** Field of view generated by a low frequency phased array or curvilinear probe.
**B.** Field of view generated by a high frequency linear probe.

The field of view is divided into near-field and far-field. Near-field structures are superficial while far-field structures are deep.

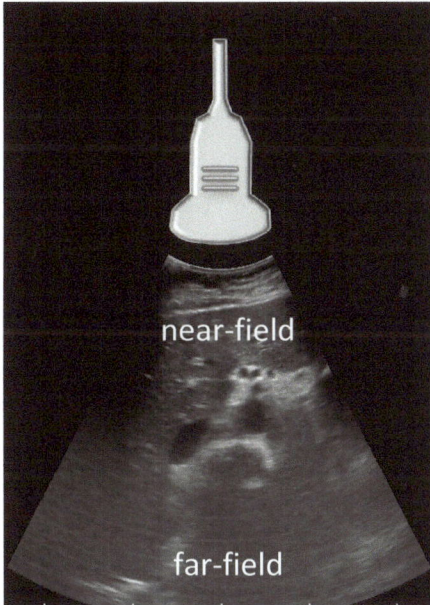

**Figure 2.8 The ultrasound image is divided into near-field and far-field.**

## Orientation of structures relative to probe position

Every probe has an orientation marker located on the side of the probe that corresponds to an orientation marker on the field of view. By noting the alignment of the orientation marker on the probe and the screen, the sonographer can keep track of where structures are situated relative to each other.

'Abdominal setting'

Consider an image of the abdomen in the transverse plane. The image is generated by placing a probe on the abdomen with the orientation marker pointing to the patient's right. The orientation marker will appear on the upper left corner of the screen. This is the convention when probes are used in the 'abdominal setting'. Therefore, structures on the patient's right appear on the left of the ultrasound field of view.

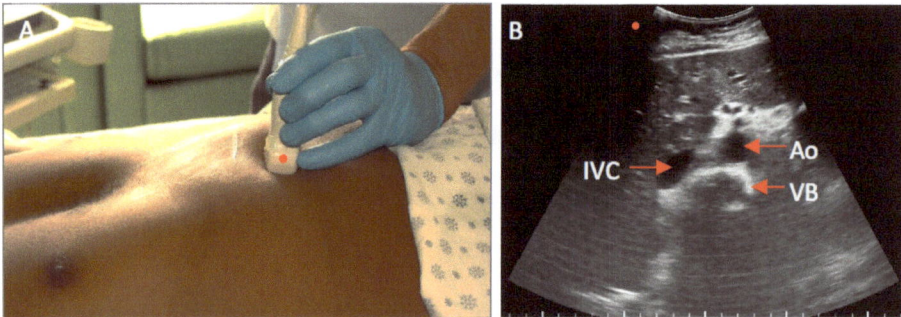

**Figure 2.9 Alignment of orientation markers on the probe and ultrasound screen.**
**A.** Imaging abdominal structures in the transverse plane with a phased array probe in the 'abdominal setting'. The orientation marker is to the patient's right.
**B.** The orientation marker appears on the upper left corner of the screen. The inferior vena cava (IVC) is to the left of the aorta (Ao) on the ultrasound screen. VB: vertebral body. Red circle denotes orientation marker.

'Cardiac setting'

Due to convention, the orientation marker will appear on the upper right hand corner of the screen when imaging the heart with any probe in the 'cardiac setting'.

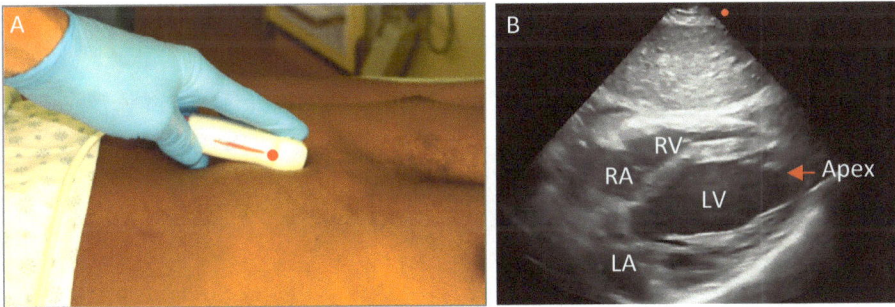

**Figure 2.10 Alignment of orientation markers on the probe and ultrasound screen for imaging the heart.**
**A.** Imaging the heart with a phased array probe in the 'cardiac setting'. The orientation marker on the probe is to the patient's left.
**B.** The orientation marker appears on the upper right corner of the screen. The apex of the heart appears on the right side of the ultrasound screen.
LV: left ventricle, LA: left atrium, RA: right atrium, RV: right ventricle. Red circle denotes orientation marker.

## 2.6 Adjustment of depth

When the structure of interest appears on the ultrasound screen, adjust the depth such that the structure appears centered in the screen (see also Figure 1.6). This adjustment will improve the quality of the image.

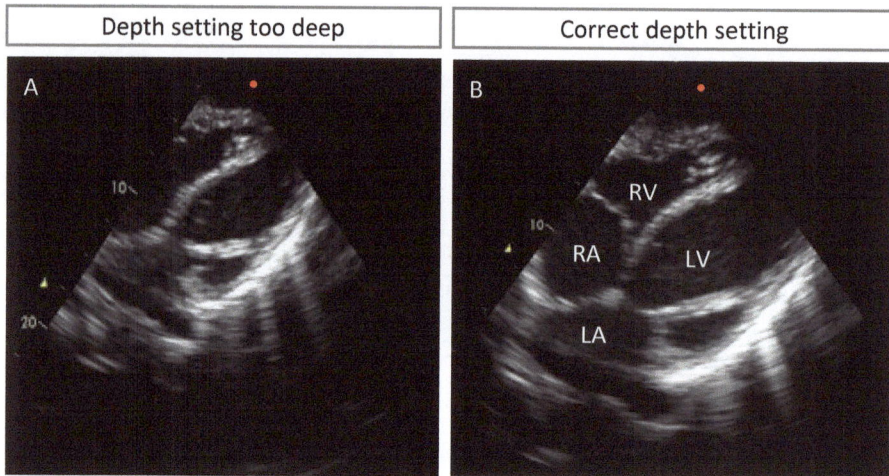

**Figure 2.11 Adjusting the depth to improve the quality of the image.**
**A.** Subxiphoid view of the heart with depth setting too deep.
**B.** Same view with correct depth setting.
LV: left ventricle, LA: left atrium, RA: right atrium, RV: right ventricle. Red circle denotes orientation marker.

## 2.7  Adjustment of gain

When gain is set too low, the image will appear dark on the screen. When gain is set too high, the image will appear white on the screen. Adjust the gain to optimize the quality of the image and improve your ability to identify structures of interest.

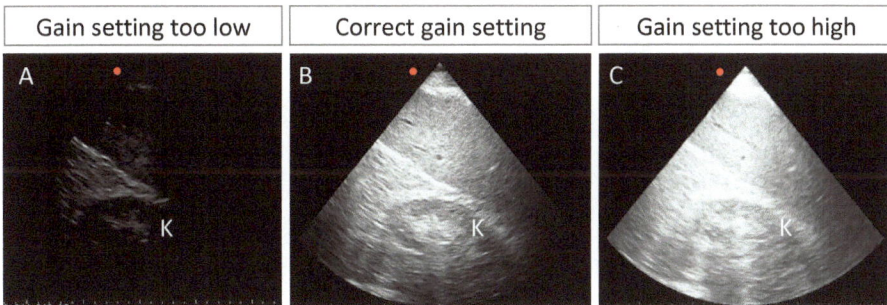

| Gain setting too low | Correct gain setting | Gain setting too high |

**Figure 2.12 Adjusting the gain to optimize the quality of the image.**
**A.** View of the kidney (K) with gain set too low.
**B.** Same kidney with correct gain setting.
**C.** Same kidney with gain set too high.
Red circle denotes orientation marker.

## 2.8 Cleaning machine and probe between patients

Since portable ultrasound machines are used on different patients, you must avoid allowing the machines to become vectors for nosocomial disease. It is imperative that the ultrasonographer follow the manufacturer's recommendations regarding the proper cleaning of the machine between patients and use gloves when examining a patient.

## 2.9 Troubleshooting tips

- To improve image quality, ensure the following are optimal:

  o patient position

  o probe choice

  o gel usage

  o gain setting

  o depth setting

  o scanning technique

- To improve image quality, it is important to orient the probe perpendicular to the structure of interest. This procedure minimizes the scatter of ultrasound and maximizes the quantity of ultrasound reflected back to the probe.

# 3. IMAGE ARTIFACTS

3.1  Common artifacts

3.2  Shadowing artifact

3.3  Enhancement artifact

3.4  Mirror image artifact

3.5  Reverberation artifact

3.6  Refraction (edge) artifact

3.7  Troubleshooting tips

## 3.1 Common artifacts

Artifacts are ultrasound images that do not represent an anatomic structure. They are generated by ultrasound interacting with structures within the body. It is important to recognize artifacts so that they are not mistaken for true structures within the body.

In this chapter we introduce five common artifacts. Each artifact offers both an advantage and disadvantage to the ultrasonographer.

## 3.2 Shadowing artifact

When ultrasound encounters high-density structures like bone or gallstones, all of the ultrasound is either absorbed by or reflected away from the surface of the structure. The surface of the structure appears hyperechoic (white). The area deep to bone or gallstones appears anechoic (black) because there is no ultrasound available deep to these structures. We call this black area a 'shadow'.

Air also causes shadowing. This is because the large difference in density between air and surrounding tissues cause the sound waves to scatter.

**Advantage**

Artifacts can be used for identifying a structure. For example, both gallbladder polyps and gallstones can appear as similar protrusions from the gallbladder wall. However, only gallstones produce a shadow deep to their image because of their high-density.

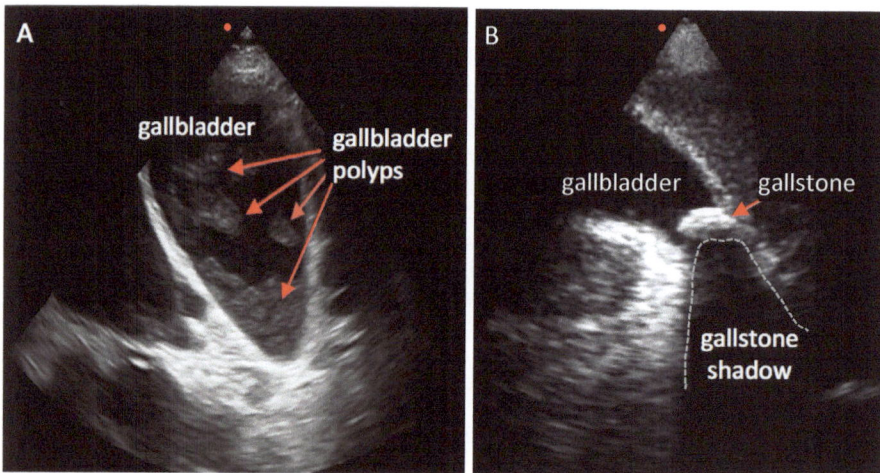

**Figure 3.1 Artifacts can be an advantage.**
**A.** An image showing gallbladder polyps. Note that the structures protruding from the gallbladder wall are not producing shadows.
**B.** This image shows a gallstone, with a characteristic dark shadow deep to the stone. Red circle denotes orientation marker.

## Disadvantage

Shadows can be a disadvantage when they obstruct the view of a deeper structure.

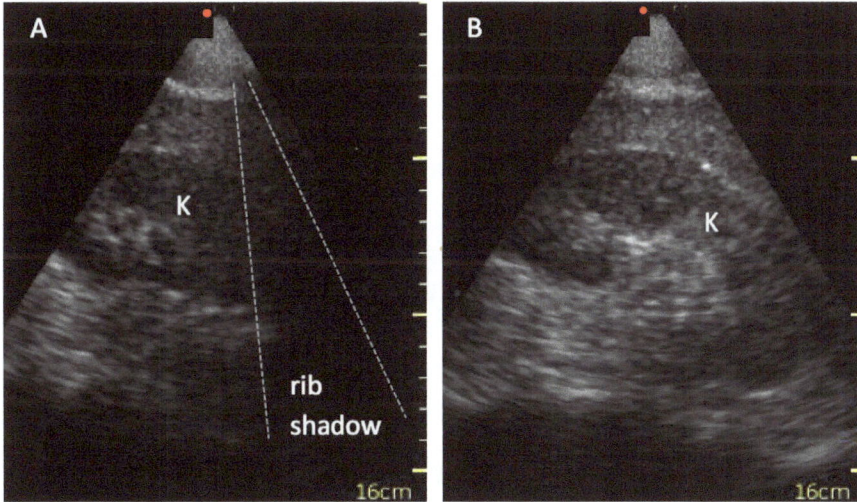

**Figure 3.2 Artifacts can be a disadvantage.**
A. Ultrasound image of the kidney (K) is obstructed by a rib shadow.
B. The rib shadow is eliminated when the same kidney is viewed from between the ribs.
Red circle denotes orientation marker.

## 3.3 Enhancement artifact

Ultrasound passes through low-density fluid filled structures, such as a gallbladder or a fluid filled cyst, with little attenuation. The ultrasound then reaches tissues deep to the fluid filled structures with more energy, making them look 'enhanced' and more echogenic (white) than surrounding tissues.

**Advantage**

An enhancement artifact can be used to differentiate between a fluid filled cyst and a tumor. Both can appear as circular structures within a solid organ. The fluid filled cyst, with its low density, will produce an enhancement artifact. The tumor, with its higher density, will produce less, if any, enhancement artifact.

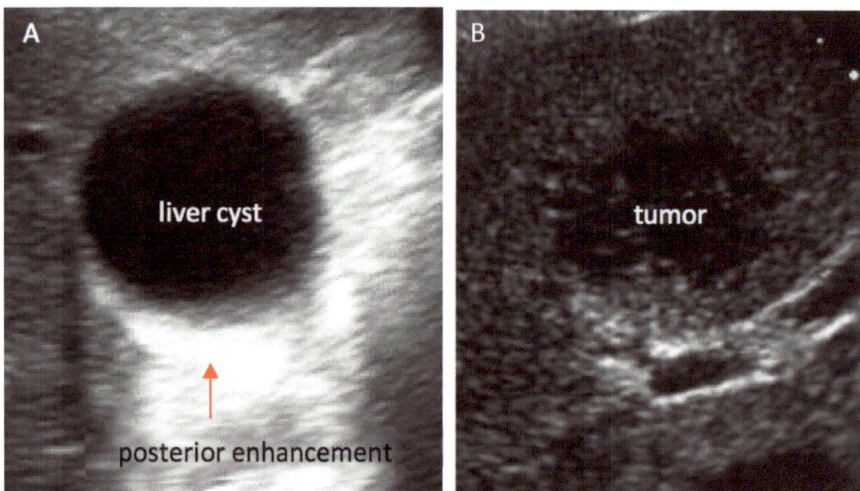

**Figure 3.3 Using enhancement artifact to identify structures.**
**A.** Ultrasound image of liver cyst demonstrating posterior enhancement artifact.
**B.** Ultrasound image of a liver tumor without posterior enhancement artifact.

**Disadvantage**

The enhancement artifact can introduce error. When measuring the thickness of the gallbladder wall, the posterior wall is 'enhanced' and appears thicker than it is. Measuring the posterior wall will overestimate the thickness of the gallbladder wall.

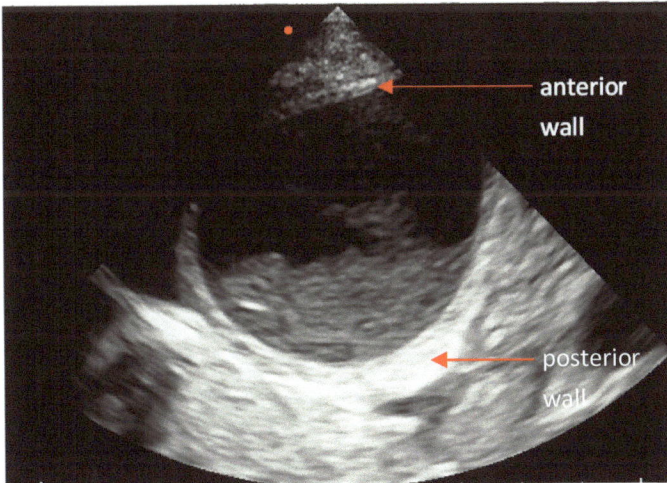

**Figure 3.4 Enhancement artifact of posterior gallbladder wall.**
Red circle denotes orientation marker.

## 3.4 Mirror image artifact

When ultrasound encounters a highly reflective curved surface such as the diaphragm, part of the reflected ultrasound travels through the liver and returns directly to the probe. However, part of the ultrasound follows a longer indirect trajectory in returning to the probe. The ultrasound machine can interpret this longer return time as representing a deeper structure. This interpretation can result in a 'mirror' image of the liver appearing deep to the diaphragm.

**Advantage**

A mirror image of the liver will not usually form in the presence of a pleural effusion. The presence of a mirror image of the liver cephalad to the diaphragm generally excludes a pleural effusion at that point.

**Disadvantage**

The mirror image of the liver can be misinterpreted as representing consolidated lung.

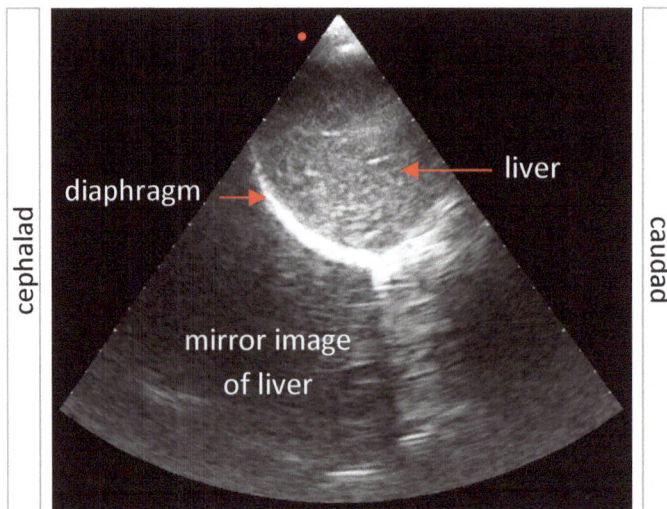

**Figure 3.5 Mirror image of the liver cephalad to the diaphragm.**
Red circle denotes orientation marker.

## 3.5 Reverberation artifact

When ultrasound encounters two closely apposed reflective surfaces, such as the parietal and visceral pleura, the ultrasound reverberates between the two surfaces. This reverberation creates parallel linear artifacts at equidistant intervals on the ultrasound image.

**Advantage**

Reverberation artifacts that occur while imaging the lung are called 'A' lines. The presence of 'A' lines on an ultrasound image of the chest can be used in the assessment of a patient with dyspnea (see Chapter 4).

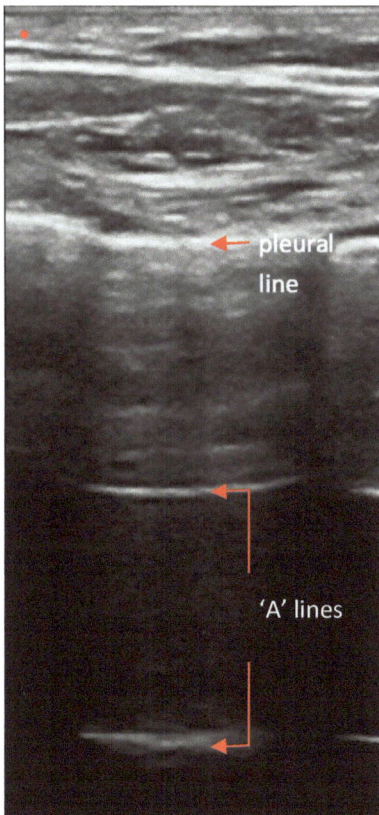

**Figure 3.6 'A' lines in a normal lung.**
Anterior chest scan with a linear probe. Red circle denotes orientation marker.

## 3.6 Refraction (edge) artifact

When ultrasound encounters the edge of a fluid filled curved structure (e.g. gallbladder), the ultrasound waves are deflected from their path. This results in an anechoic (black) artifact that projects from the edge of the fluid filled structure and extends into the far-field.

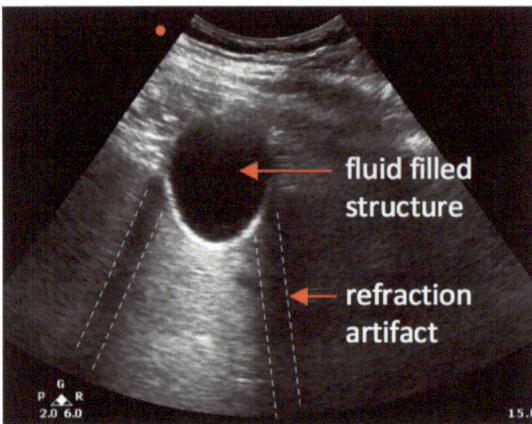

**Figure 3.7 Refraction (edge) artifact surrounding a fluid filled structure.**
Red circle denotes orientation marker.

## 3.7 Troubleshooting tips

- When rib shadows obscure the view of the kidney, ask the patient to breathe in and hold their breath. This action will cause the kidney to descend below the ribs and improve the quality of the image. By moving the probe caudally, the kidney can now be imaged without being impeded by the rib

- The enhancement artifact overestimates the thickness of the posterior gallbladder wall. Therefore, measure the thickness of the anterior gallbladder wall instead

- Mirror image artifacts generally disappear when the orientation of the probe is changed

- Reverberation artifacts ('A' lines) appear more curved when using a curvilinear or phased array probe.

# 4. DYSPNEA

4.1  Probe choice

4.2  Patient position and scanning technique-Anterior chest exam

4.3  Lung sliding

4.4  'A' lines

4.5  'B' lines

4.6  Lung profiles

4.7  Posterolateral chest exam

4.8  Troubleshooting tips

4.9  False-positives and false-negatives

4.10  CPoCUS documentation standards

**Case scenario:**

A 70 year old woman presents herself to your clinic complaining of dyspnea. She is too short of breath to provide a useful history. Her respiratory rate is 40 breaths/min, her oxygen saturation is 80%, and she is tachycardic with normal blood pressure. On auscultation, there is poor air entry bilaterally.

**Impression:**

Dyspnea, not yet determined. Consider common causes.

Common causes of **dyspnea** can be recognized by ultrasound examination of the chest. This chapter reviews the technique for diagnosis of pneumothorax, interpretation of lung artifacts, and identification of pleural effusions.

## 4.1 Probe choice

Both low and high frequency probes can be used for this application.

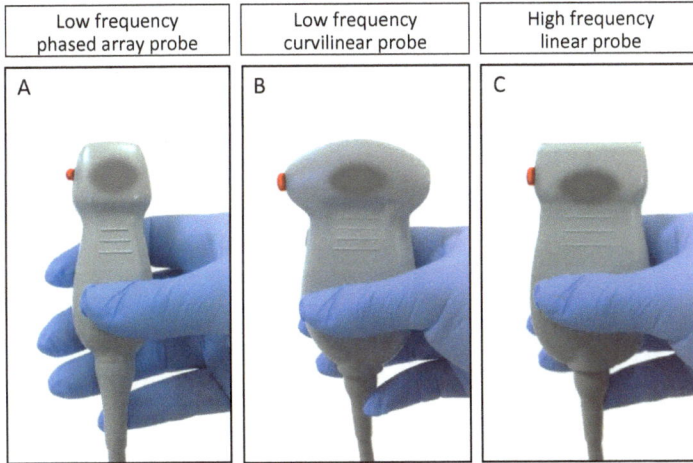

**Figure 4.1 Low and high frequency probes that can be used for assessing a patient with dyspnea.**
**A.** Phased array probe (low frequency).
**B.** Curvilinear probe (low frequency).
**C.** Linear probe (high frequency).
Red circle denotes orientation marker.

## 4.2 Patient position and scanning technique-
## Anterior chest exam

The patient should lie supine or be semi-seated in bed depending on the clinical indication. Scan the most anterior part of the chest in the mid-clavicular line (approximately 4^th interspace). Then proceed to scan the anterior chest in three different interspaces in the mid-clavicular line on both sides.

Scanning should be performed in the sagittal plane so that the ribs and rib shadows can be used as landmarks.

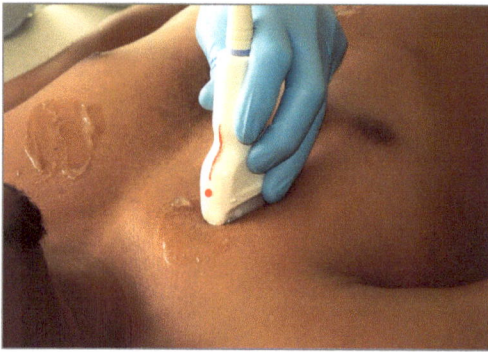

**Figure 4.2 Scanning technique for imaging the anterior chest.**
The anterior chest is imaged bilaterally with a linear probe in the mid-clavicular line. The orientation marker points cephalad.

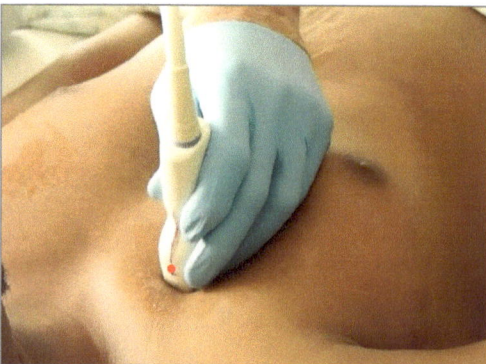

**Video 4.1 Scanning technique with lateral rocking motion.**
The lateral rocking motion of the probe improves the sensitivity for locating pathology [3]. Video: bedsideultrasoundlevel1.com

## 4.3 Lung sliding

During respiration, the parietal and visceral pleura slide over one another. This horizontal pleural movement during respiration is observed on an ultrasound image and is called **lung sliding** [4].

### Characteristics of lung sliding

- The area deep to the pleural line sways side-to-side with the patient's breathing

- The hyperechoic (white) pleural line moves or 'shimmers'

### Clinical relevance - Pneumothorax

### Ruling out pneumothorax

A pneumothorax is a collection of air between the parietal and visceral pleura. Air in the pleural space prevents the contact between the pleurae and therefore prevents lung sliding. In all cases of pneumothorax, lung sliding will be absent in the scanned area over the anterior chest of a supine patient. Therefore, normal lung sliding confidently rules out pneumothorax [5-8].

Two other findings rule out pneumothorax. The presence of **'B' lines** (see Section 4.5) rules out a pneumothorax at the location of the scan. This is because for 'B' lines to form, the visceral and parietal pleura must be in contact with one another. In a pneumothorax there is air between the visceral and parietal pleura, so 'B' lines cannot form. A **lung pulse** is a pulsation seen on the pleural line, even when a patient is not breathing. It is caused by transmission of the heart contractions through intact lung. When air is trapped between the visceral and parietal pleura in a pneumothorax, the lung pulse is not seen. Therefore, either **'B' lines** or a **lung pulse** on the scan of the anterior chest of a supine patient rule out pneumothorax.

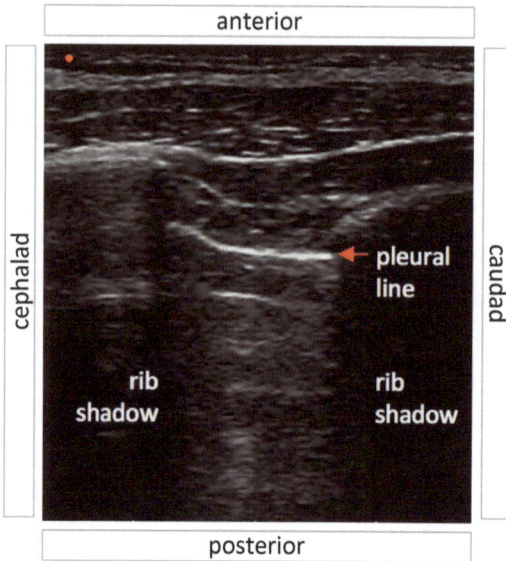

**Video 4.2 Presence of lung sliding on the anterior chest using a linear probe.**
The hyperechoic (white) pleural line 'shimmers', thus illustrating lung sliding.
Accordingly, this patient does not have a pneumothorax.
Video: bedsideultrasoundlevel1.com

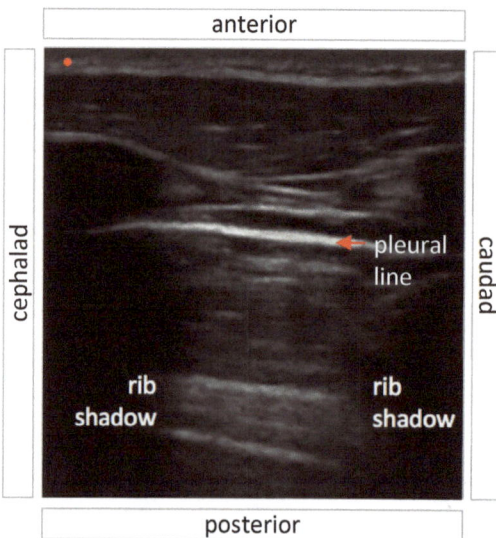

**Video 4.3 Lung pulse.**
Note that lung sliding is absent but a pulsation of the pleural line (lung pulse) is
appreciated. Video: bedsideultrasoundlevel1.com

## Ruling in pneumothorax

Importantly, the absence of lung sliding **suggests but is not specific** for a pneumothorax because there are other conditions in which lung sliding is absent or hard to detect. These conditions include pleural adhesions, atelectasis, apnea, unilateral bronchial intubation, and extremely shallow rapid breathing (asthma) [3].

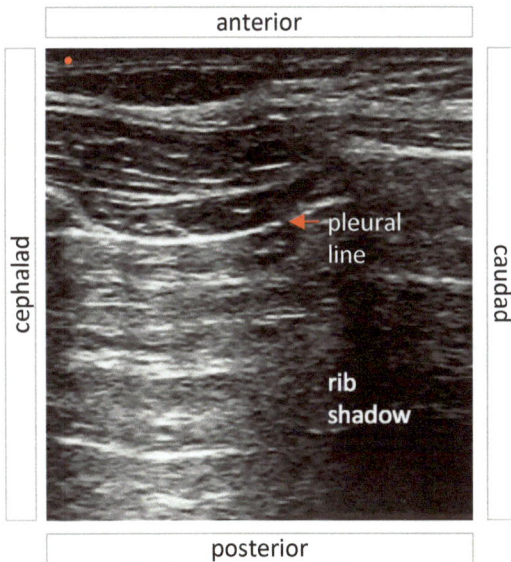

**Video 4.4**
**Absence of lung sliding on the anterior chest using a linear probe.**
Note that the pleural line does not 'shimmer' or slide laterally. Therefore, this patient may have a pneumothorax. Video: bedsideultrasoundlevel1.com

When the absence of lung sliding is observed, a pneumothorax can be confirmed by detecting a **lung point**. The lung point is an ultrasound landmark specific for a pneumothorax [9].

To look for a lung point, start scanning the anterior chest of a supine patient in whom you have detected the absence of lung sliding. Gradually scan over the chest posterolaterally. A lung point occurs at the point where the visceral and parietal pleurae separate to form the pneumothorax. It can be observed as the alternating presence and absence of lung sliding between two ribs as the patient breathes.

The presence of a lung point confirms a pneumothorax on the side of the chest being imaged.

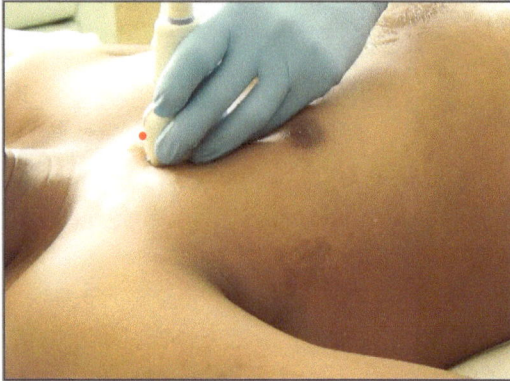

**Video 4.5 Scanning technique for imaging a lung point using a linear probe.**
Video: bedsideultrasoundlevel1.com

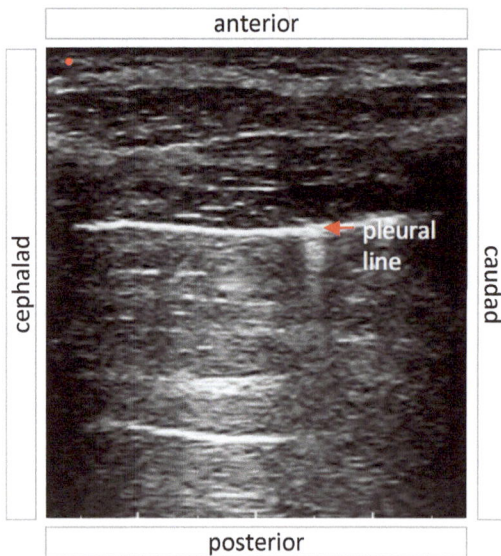

**Video 4.6 Lung point on posterolateral chest using linear probe.**
Note the lung sliding coming and going from the right of the screen.
Video: bedsideultrasoundlevel1.com

**Pitfalls in diagnosing pneumothorax**

The **cardiac lung point** and the **liver lung point** are two normal findings which can mimic a lung point. When scanning the left chest, the image of the heart may extend into the ultrasound image. The intersection between lung sliding and the pericardium is called a cardiac lung point and can mimic a lung point. When scanning the right chest, the liver lung point occurs as the patient breathes out and the edge of the liver moves into the ultrasound image. The intersection between lung sliding and the liver capsule is called the liver lung point and can mimic a lung point.

Patients with pneumothorax can develop subcutaneous emphysema (air trapped within the subcutaneous tissues). In subcutaneous emphysema, there are multiple comet tail artifacts extending from the subcutaneous tissues *above* the pleural line. These **'E' lines** can obscure the ultrasound image of the pleural line and make it difficult to determine whether lung sliding is present.

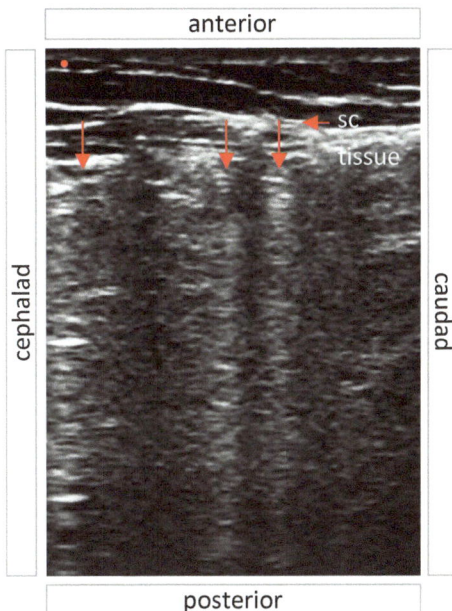

**Figure 4.3 'E' lines in a patient with subcutaneous emphysema.**
Note multiple hyperechoic comet tail artifacts (downward arrows) originating in the subcutaneous (sc) tissues.

## 4.4 'A' lines

An **'A' line** artifact is a hyperechoic (white) horizontal line arising at regular intervals from the pleural line. An 'A' line artifact is produced when scanning the anterior chest of a patient with normal lungs or in a patient with diseased lungs without interstitial disease (e.g. obstructive airways disease, pulmonary embolism) [10].

**Characteristics of 'A' lines**

- Horizontal hyperechoic (white) lines
- Evenly spaced throughout the ultrasound field
- Immobile

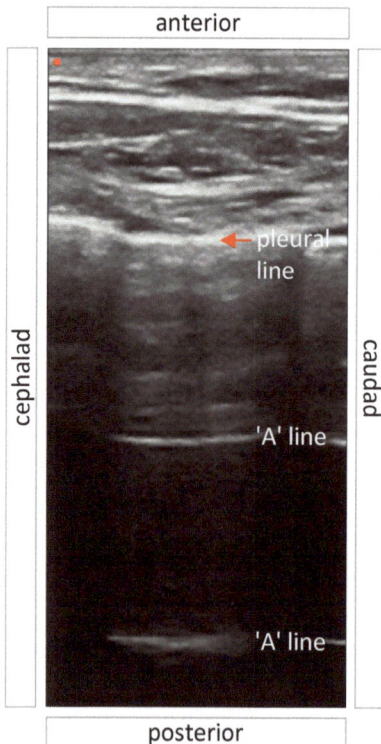

**Figure 4.4 'A' lines in a normal lung.**
Anterior chest scan with a linear probe.

## 4.5 'B' lines

A **'B' line** artifact is a hyperechoic (white) vertical line arising from the pleural line. 'B' lines are sometimes referred to as 'comet tail artifacts'. A 'B' line is a non-specific artifact produced with any disease of the pulmonary interstitium including pneumonia, pulmonary edema, interstitial fibrosis, and acute respiratory distress syndrome. Three or more 'B' lines between two rib shadows are considered abnormal [11].

### Characteristics of 'B' lines

- Vertical, comet-shaped hyperechoic (white) lines

- Originate at the pleural line and extend to the far-field of the ultrasound screen

- Move with the pleural line

- Eliminate 'A' lines

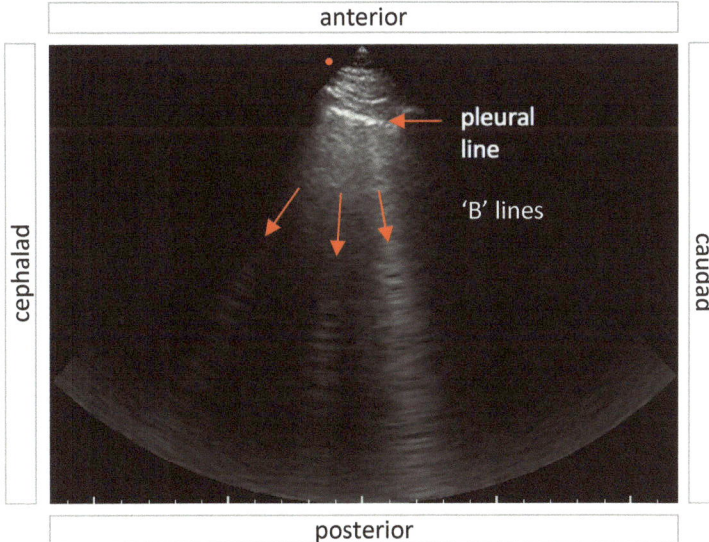

**Video 4.7 'B' lines in a diseased lung.**
Anterior chest scan (with a phased array probe in the abdominal setting) displaying vertical 'B' lines that originate at the pleural line and extend to the far-field.
Video: bedsideultrasoundlevel1.com

## 4.6 Lung profiles

### Clinical relevance - 'A' profile

If you see lung sliding with 'A' lines on bilateral anterior chest exams, the patient is defined as having an **'A' profile.** Patients presenting with dyspnea and an 'A' profile generally have chronic obstructive pulmonary disease (COPD) or asthma exacerbation. Patients with dyspnea, an 'A' profile, and a deep venous thrombosis (DVT) are likely to have a pulmonary embolism [12].

### Clinical relevance - 'B' profile

If you see lung sliding with 'B' lines on bilateral anterior chest scans, the patient is defined as having a **'B' profile**. Patients with a 'B' profile have interstitial pulmonary pathology. In patients presenting with dyspnea to the emergency room, this is most likely due to pulmonary edema [12].

However, the interpretation of lung profiles must always be done in context of the clinical impression. For example, a patient presenting with a 'B' profile in association with fever, rigors, cough, and productive sputum, likely has bilateral pneumonia and not cardiogenic pulmonary edema.

### Clinical relevance - 'AB' profile

If one side of the anterior chest has 'A' lines while the other side has 'B' lines the patient is said to have an **'AB' profile.** Patients presenting with an 'AB' profile and dyspnea are likely to have pneumonia as the cause of their dyspnea [12].

**Table 4.1 Lung profiles and common associated pathologies in outpatients presenting with dyspnea**

| Lung profile | Pathology |
|---|---|
| 'A' profile 'A' lines   'A' lines | COPD<br>Asthma<br>Pulmonary embolism (if DVT present) |
| 'B' profile 'B' lines   'B' lines | Interstitial pathology<br>e.g. cardiogenic pulmonary edema |
| 'AB' profile 'A' lines   'B' lines | Pneumonia |

## 4.7 Posterolateral chest exam

The posterolateral chest is examined for **pleural effusions** and **lung consolidation**. It is also useful for confirming diaphragmatic function. The patient should be scanned semi-seated in bed. Place the probe in the coronal plane on the posterior axillary line at the level of the xiphoid process.

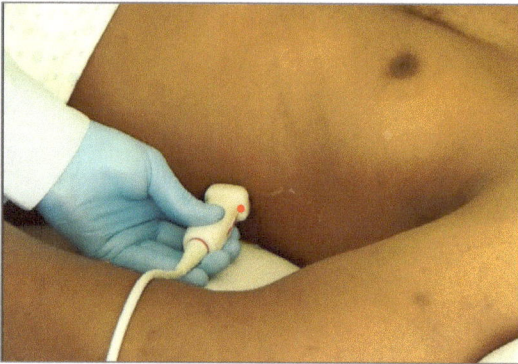

**Video 4.8 Scanning technique for imaging a pleural effusion or lung consolidation over the left posterolateral chest.**
Video:
bedsideultrasoundlevel1.com

### Characteristics of the posterolateral chest exam

- Diaphragm appears as a hyperechoic (white) line, concave caudally that descends (moves caudally) during inspiration

- Normal lung appears as a **curtain sign** sweeping into the field as the diaphragm descends.

## Clinical relevance - Pleural effusion and lung consolidation

- Pleural effusion is a collection of fluid between the parietal and visceral pleura

- Pleural effusion appears as an anechoic (black) area above the diaphragm. Pleural effusions that contain hyperechoic (white) floating particles or septae are likely to be exudative [13]. Normally the thoracic spine is not visible cephalad to the diaphragm due to the scattering of ultrasound when it contacts air filled lung tissue. When a pleural effusion or consolidated lung is present, these pathologies act as an acoustic window allowing ultrasound to travel through and visualize the thoracic spine cephalad to the diaphragm. When the thoracic spine is visualized cephalad to the diaphragm it is called the **spine sign**. The spine sign indicates there is an acoustic window (pleural effusion or consolidated lung) cephalad to the diaphragm

- Lung consolidation appears as a hypoechoic (grey) structure above the diaphragm

- Patients with dyspnea, a normal anterior chest exam (bilateral 'A' lines), no DVT, and an unilateral pleural effusion or consolidation likely have pneumonia [12]

- Patients with dyspnea, left ventricular dysfunction, a 'B' profile, and bilateral pleural effusions likely have congestive heart failure [12]

- A diaphragm that ascends during inspiration suggests diaphragmatic paralysis or fatigue (correlate to the clinical syndrome of paradoxical breathing).

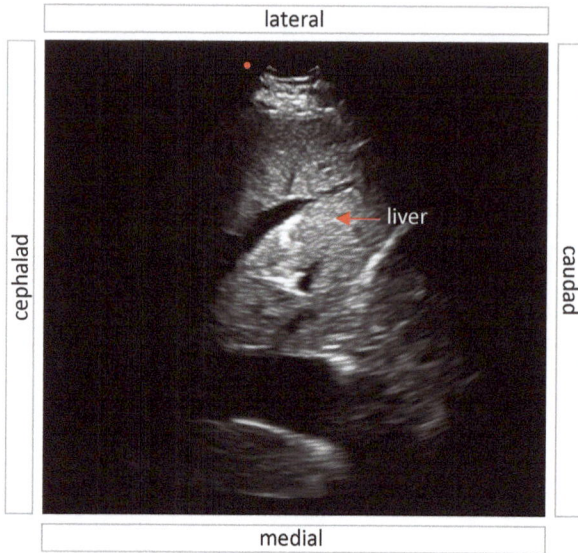

**Video 4.9 Normal lung revealed by a posterolateral chest scan with a phased array probe in the abdominal setting.**
As the diaphragm descends caudally, the lung enters the left-side field of view. This is termed the 'curtain' sign. Video: bedsideultrasoundlevel1.com

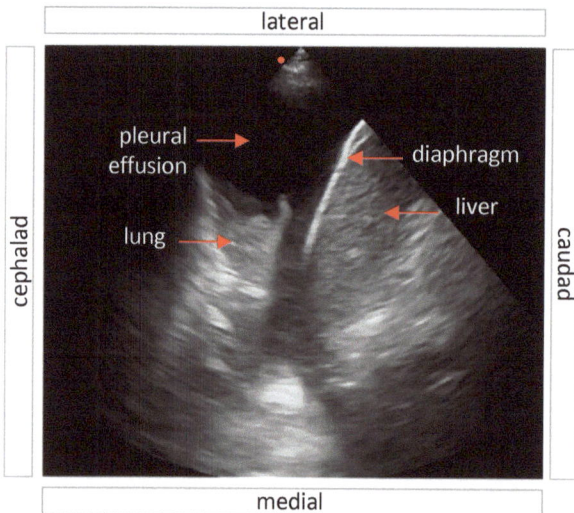

**Video 4.10 Large pleural effusion revealed by a posterolateral chest scan with a phased array probe in the abdominal setting.**
The pleural effusion is cephalad to the diaphragm and appears anechoic (black).
Video: bedsideultrasoundlevel1.com

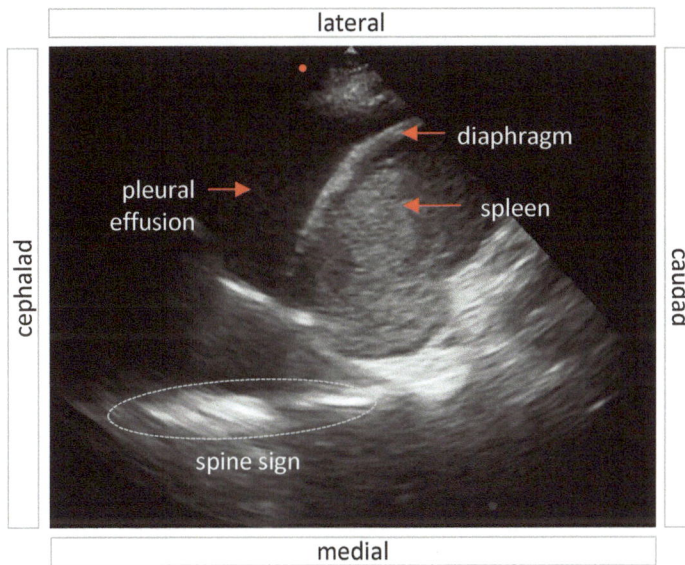

**Figure 4.5 Spine sign revealed by a posterolateral chest scan with a phased array probe in the abdominal setting.**

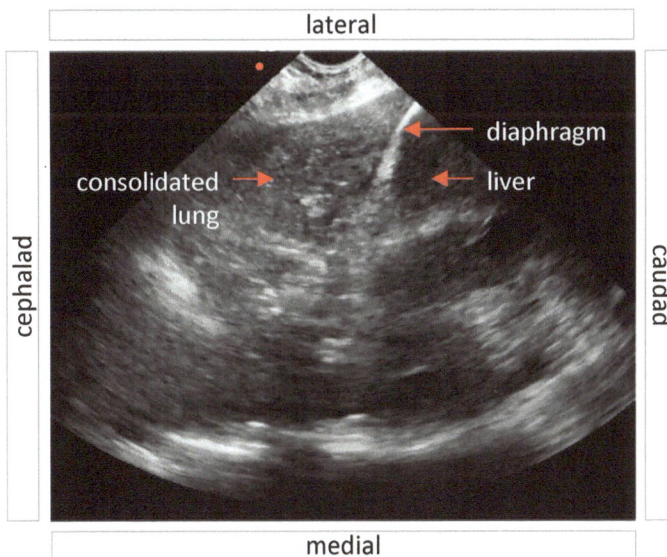

**Figure 4.6 Lung consolidation revealed by a posterolateral chest scan with a phased array probe in the abdominal setting.**
The consolidated lung is a hypoechoic (grey) structure.

## 4.8 Troubleshooting tips

- To detect a pneumothorax in a supine patient, be sure to examine the anterior chest at the mid-clavicular line in three separate intercostal spaces

- Beware that a lung point will not be found in a tension pneumothorax because the lung is completely collapsed in this condition and therefore does not contact the chest wall

- In cachectic patients with a protruding rib cage, it is difficult to establish adequate contact between a linear probe and the chest wall. This difficulty can be overcome by turning the probe in the transverse plane so that it fits between the ribs, or by using a microconvex probe

- Sometimes, lung sliding is difficult to identify with a low frequency probe due to its relatively low resolution. In this case, use a high frequency linear probe instead.

## 4.9 False-positives and false-negatives

**False-positives:**

- **Lung point:** The cardiac lung point and the liver lung points can mimic a lung point and are therefore false-positives for a lung point

- **'B' lines:** 'E' lines, seen in subcutaneous emphysema, can mimic 'B' lines and are thus false-positives for 'B' lines.

## 4.10 CPoCUS documentation standards

The Canadian Point of Care Ultrasound Society (CPoCUS) recommends that POCUS exams be documented as follows:

- **Pneumothorax (PTX):**
  o  Negative study:   PTX -
  o  Positive study:   PTX +
  o  Indeterminate:   PTX indeterminate
- **Pleural effusion:**
  o  Negative study:   pleural effusion –
  o  Positive study:   pleural effusion +
  o  Indeterminate:   pleural effusion indeterminate

**Case closed:**

The 70 year old woman who presented herself to your clinic complaining of dyspnea has clinical evidence of congestive heart failure. She is found to have a 'B' profile on lung ultrasound. Diuretic is administered, and the patient is hospitalized.

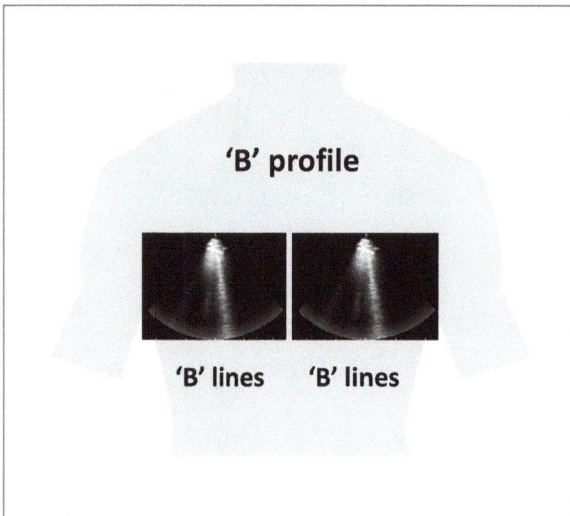

**Figure 4.7 Patient with a 'B' profile has 'B' lines on bilateral anterior chest scans.**

# 5. UNDIFFERENTIATED HYPOTENSION

5.1  Probe choice

5.2  Patient position and scanning technique

5.3  Left ventricular function

5.4  Right to left ventricular diameter ratio

5.5  Pericardial effusion

5.6  Volume status and the IVC

5.7  Additional ultrasound assessments for hypotension

5.8  Troubleshooting tips

5.9  False-positives and false-negatives

5.10  CPoCUS documentation standards

**Case scenario:**

An 80 year old man is found unconscious in his home, and no medical history is available. At the hospital, he is hypotensive with a blood pressure of 70/40 mmHg, and a heart rate of 120 beats/min. He is normothermic, breathing shallowly at 30 breaths/min, and his oxygen saturation is unobtainable. His neck veins are not visible. He has poor air entry bilaterally and some tenderness on abdominal exam. No bowel sounds are present. His legs are mottled.

**Impression:**

Undifferentiated hypotension. Consider common causes.

Bedside ultrasound can help to identify certain causes of **undifferentiated hypotension**. This chapter introduces the ultrasonographic signs associated with left ventricular dysfunction, massive pulmonary embolism, tamponade, and hypovolemia.

## 5.1 Probe choice

A low frequency phased array probe is commonly used for this application, however a low frequency curvilinear probe is also an appropriate choice.

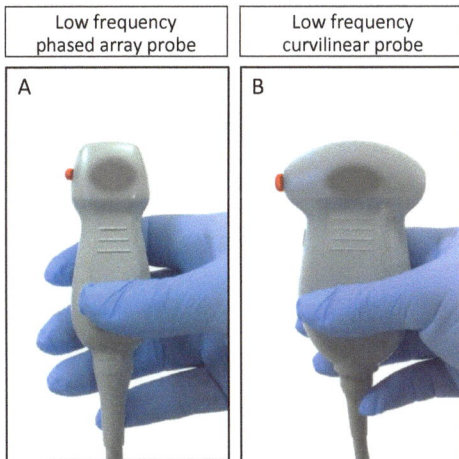

**Figure 5.1 Low frequency probes that can be used for assessing a patient with undifferentiated hypotension.**
**A.** A phased array probe.
**B.** A curvilinear probe.
Red circle denotes orientation marker.

## 5.2 Patient position and scanning technique

This application is best performed with the patient in the supine position.

## 5.3 Left ventricular function

Estimating left ventricular (LV) function can help distinguish between different causes of hypotension. To estimate LV function, obtain a subxiphoid view of the heart by placing the probe on the abdomen between the umbilicus and the xiphoid area as shown (Video 5.1). If using the phased array probe in the cardiac setting, the orientation marker points to the patient's left side. If the probe is in the abdominal setting, the orientation marker points to the patient's right side. Regardless of the setting, the image on the screen is identical. The liver will appear in the near-field. The liver acts as an acoustic window through which you can image the heart.

If you are having trouble obtaining a subxiphoid image:

- Ask the patient to bend their knees to relax their abdominal musculature

- Ask the patient to breathe in and hold their breath. This action can bring the heart closer to the probe and provide a better image

- Move the probe to the patient's right side. Sometimes the image improves due to the liver acting as an acoustic window.

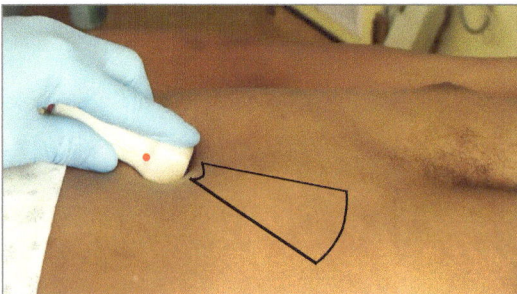

**Video 5.1 Scanning technique to obtain a subxiphoid view of the heart.**
Video:
bedsideultrasoundlevel1.com

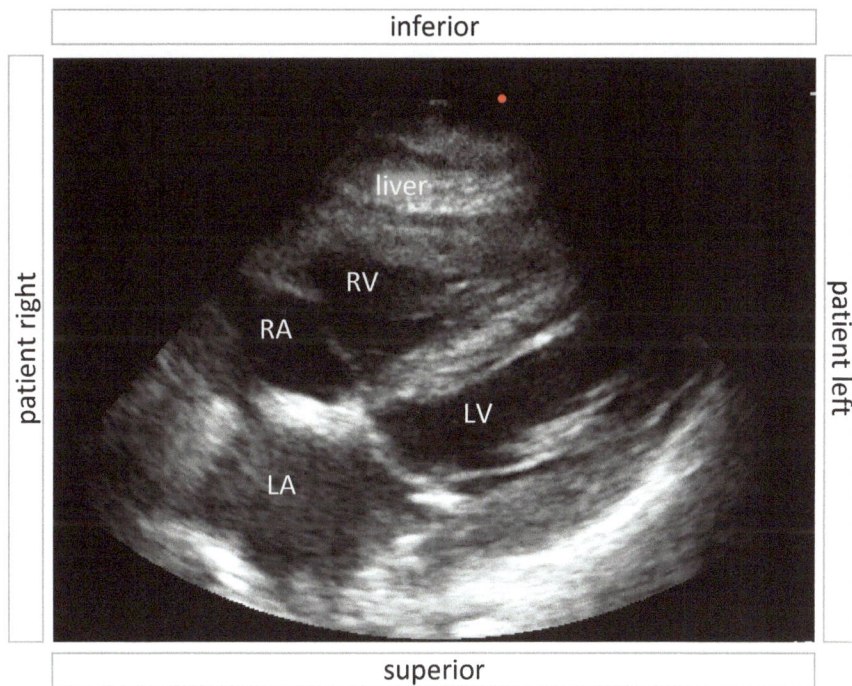

**Figure 5.2 Subxiphoid view of the heart.**
Subxiphoid view of the heart using a phased array probe in the cardiac setting.
LV: left ventricle, LA: left atrium, RA: right atrium, RV: right ventricle.

On the ultrasound image of a normal heart during systole, the LV walls thicken, and the LV diameter decreases by 30%. The LV diameter is measured from inner wall to inner wall. The measurement is made one third of the way from the mitral valve annulus to the apex. The decrease in LV diameter during systole is termed **'fractional shortening'** [14].

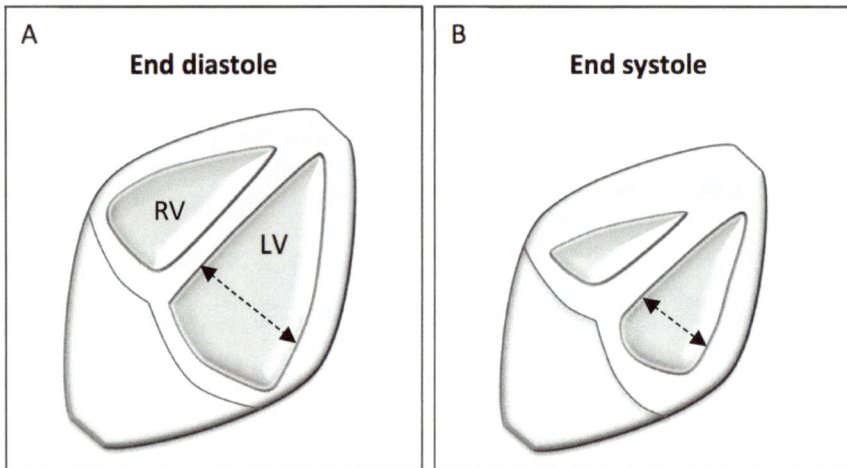

**Figure 5.3 Measuring left ventricular (LV) diameter.**
LV diameter is measured from inner wall to inner wall.
**A.** LV diameter at the end of diastole.
**B.** LV diameter decreases by 30% during normal systole.
RV: Right ventricle.

LV function can also be assessed using a subjective visual estimate of the change in LV size between systole and diastole [15-18].

The following four videos illustrate different categories of LV function.

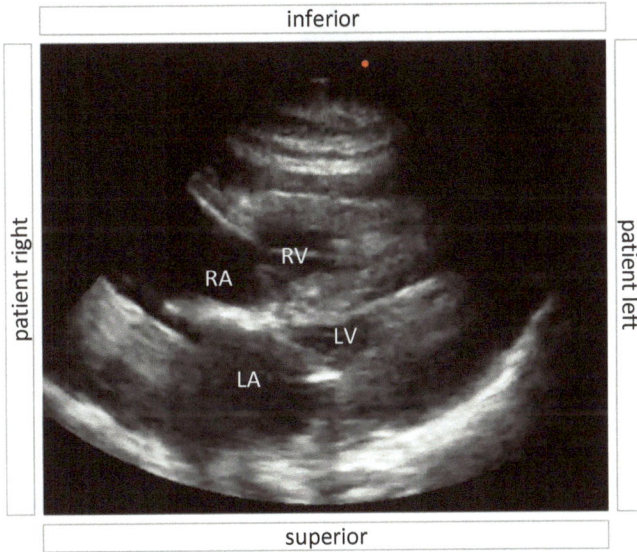

**Video 5.2 Hyperdynamic LV function in the subxiphoid view.**
LV: left ventricle, LA: left atrium, RA: right atrium, RV: right ventricle.
Video: bedsideultrasoundlevel1.com

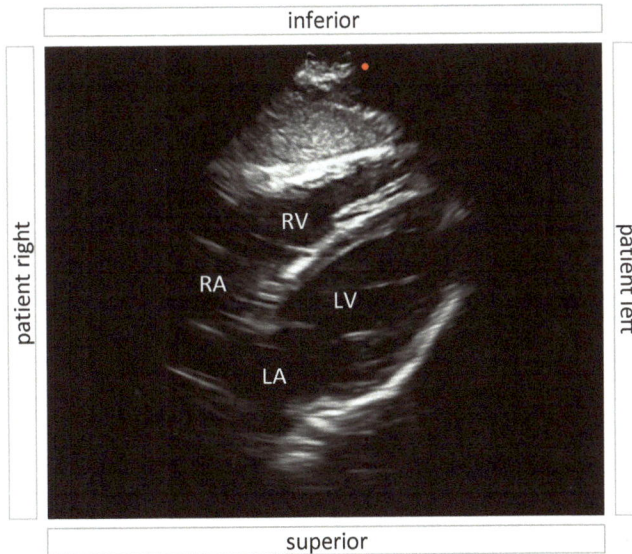

**Video 5.3 Normal LV function in the subxiphoid view.**
LV: left ventricle, LA: left atrium, RA: right atrium, RV: right ventricle.
Video: bedsideultrasoundlevel1.com

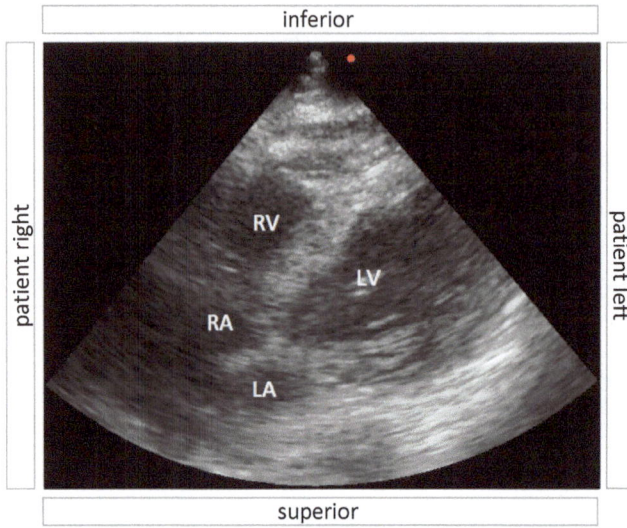

**Video 5.4 Moderate LV dysfunction in the subxiphoid view.**
LV: left ventricle, LA: left atrium, RA: right atrium, RV: right ventricle.
Video: bedsideultrasoundlevel1.com

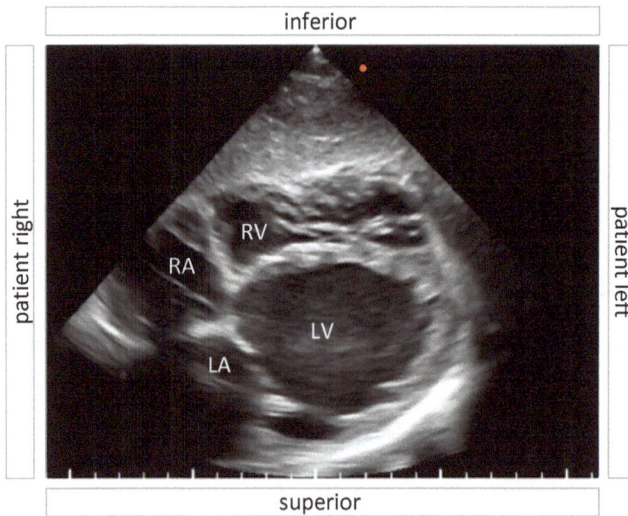

**Video 5.5 Severe LV dysfunction in the subxiphoid view.**
LV: left ventricle, LA: left atrium, RA: right atrium, RV: right ventricle.
Video: bedsideultrasoundlevel1.com

**Summary:** LV function can be classified into three categories: hyperdynamic, normal, and LV dysfunction (mild, moderate, and severe).

**Table 5.1 Categories and characteristics of left ventricular (LV) function**

| Categories of LV function | Ultrasound image characteristics |
|---|---|
| Hyperdynamic LV function | Tachycardia<br><br>Thickening of ventricular walls during systole<br><br>Fractional shortening of LV diameter greater than 30% during systole |
| Normal LV function | Thickening of ventricular walls during systole<br><br>Fractional shortening of LV diameter by 30% during systole |
| LV dysfunction (mild, moderate, and severe) | Progressive decreases in:<br>• wall thickening during systole<br>• wall motion during systole<br>• fractional shortening of LV diameter during systole |

## Clinical relevance - LV dysfunction

In a hypotensive patient:

- Hyperdynamic LV function is consistent with hypovolemia as a cause of the hypotension (e.g. bleeding) among other diagnoses (Table 5.2)

- Moderate and severe LV dysfunction are consistent with a cardiogenic cause for the hypotension (e.g. myocardial infarction).

## 5.4 Right to left ventricular diameter ratio

Normally the right ventricular (RV) chamber diameter should not exceed 60% of the LV chamber diameter at the end of diastole. Thus the RV to LV diameter ratio should not exceed 0.6 (RV:LV ratio ≤ 0.6) [19]. RV chamber diameter is measured from inner wall to inner wall [14].

The RV diameter increases acutely with massive pulmonary emboli due to an abrupt rise in the right ventricular afterload [20].

### Clinical relevance - Pulmonary embolism

In a hypotensive patient with a suspected pulmonary embolism:

- An acute increase in the RV:LV ratio supports the suspicion of a pulmonary embolism as a cause of hypotension

- A normal RV:LV ratio does not rule out pulmonary embolism, but makes massive pulmonary embolism as the sole cause of hypotension unlikely.

Caution is warranted before attributing an increased RV:LV ratio to pulmonary embolism. An increase in the RV:LV ratio can be seen in other acute (pneumonia, acute respiratory distress syndrome) and chronic (chronic obstructive pulmonary disease) conditions [21].

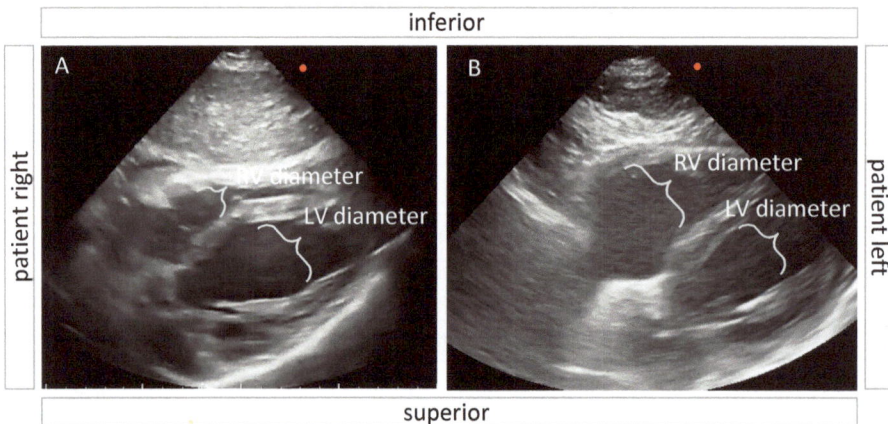

**Figure 5.4 Right to left ventricular diameter ratio in a subxiphoid view of the heart.**
**A.** Normal right ventricular (RV) to left ventricular (LV) diameter ratio (≤ 0.6).
**B.** Increased RV:LV (>0.6).

## 5.5 Pericardial effusion

A pericardial effusion is a collection of fluid between the parietal and visceral pericardium. A pericardial effusion will appear as an anechoic (black) area in the infero-posterior region of the heart. The inferior region of the heart is the wall of the right ventricle visible in the near-field of the subxiphoid view. It is necessary to image the right ventricular wall until it intersects with the interventricular septum. Once the inferior heart is identified, the inferior pericardium should be swept completely anterior and posterior to look for pericardial effusion.

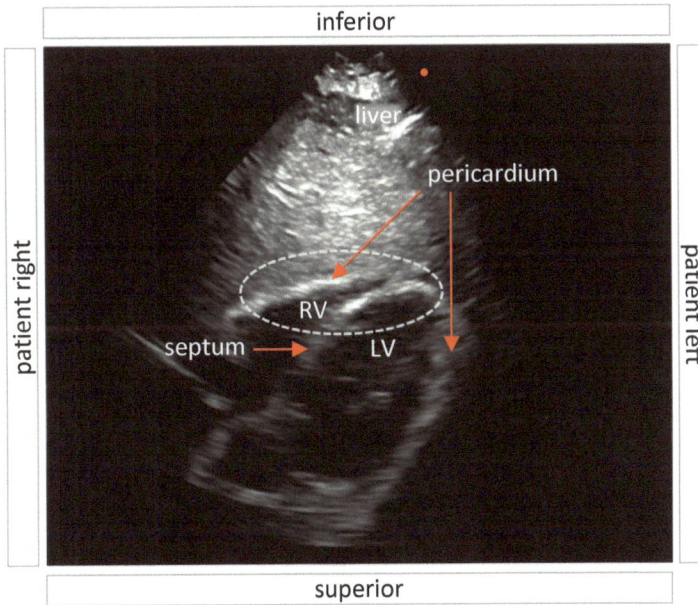

**Figure 5.5 Subxiphoid view of the heart showing the inferior pericardium (dashed area) that must be scanned to assess for pericardial effusion.**
LV: left ventricle, RV: right ventricle.

**Clinical relevance - Cardiac tamponade**

When a pericardial effusion reduces heart chamber compliance and leads to a decrease in venous return, cardiac output, and blood pressure, this is termed **cardiac tamponade** [20].

In a hypotensive patient:

- The presence of a pericardial effusion raises the possibility that cardiac tamponade is present. Note that cardiac tamponade is a clinical diagnosis. In patients whose pericardial effusion has developed slowly, significant pericardial effusions can be present without hemodynamic compromise and tamponade. Conversely, when fluid accumulates quickly (as in trauma), hemodynamic compromise can occur even with small pericardial effusions

- The absence of pericardial effusion excludes cardiac tamponade.

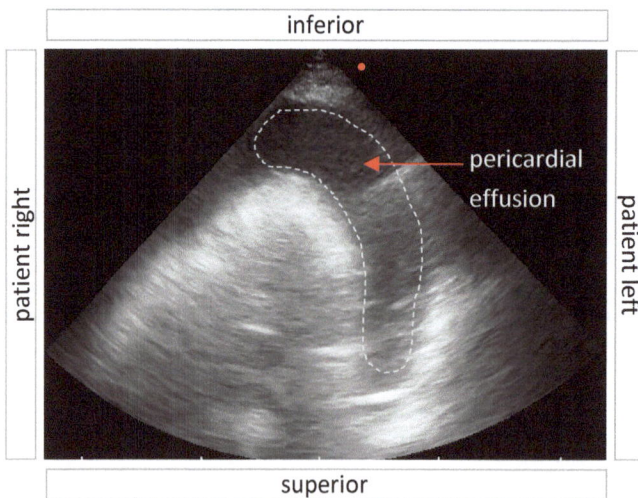

**Video 5.6 A large pericardial effusion in the subxiphoid view.**
The heart chambers are collapsed due to the pericardial effusion. This patient has tamponade. Video: bedsideultrasoundlevel1.com

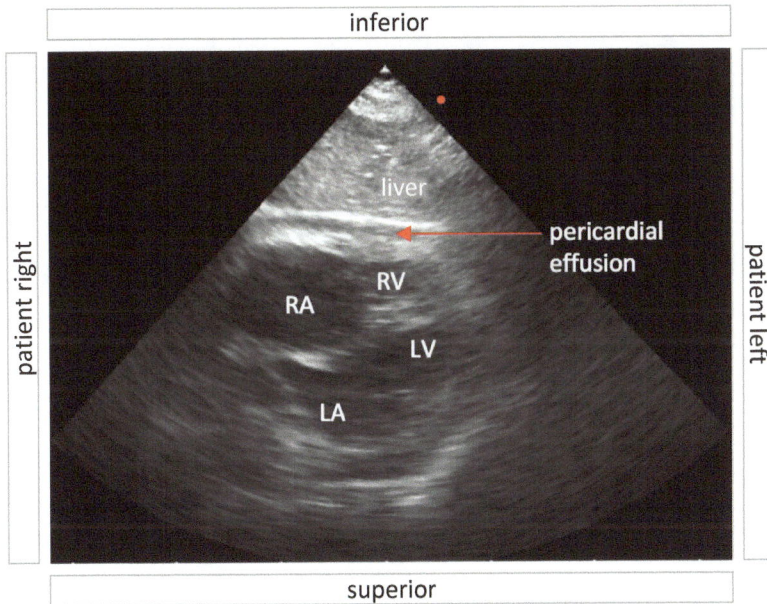

**Figure 5.6 Small pericardial effusion in the subxiphoid view.**
A pericardial fat pad was ruled out. LV: left ventricle, LA: left atrium, RA: right atrium, RV: right ventricle.

## 5.6 Volume status and the IVC

Vascular volume depletion (**hypovolemia**) is one of the causes of hypotension. Volume status can be grossly assessed with ultrasound imaging of the diameter of the inferior vena cava (IVC) and its respiratory variability.

Respiratory variability of the IVC describes the variation in IVC diameter as the patient breathes. The variability is caused by changes in intrathoracic pressure during respiration.

The diameter and respiratory variability of the IVC are measured 3-4 cm proximal to the right atrial-IVC junction [22-24].

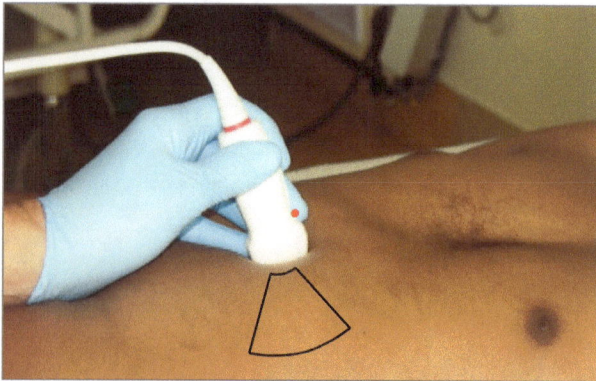

**Figure 5.7 Scanning technique for imaging the inferior vena cava (IVC).**
A phased array probe is placed in the subxiphoid area with the orientation marker pointing cephalad to image the IVC in the sagittal plane.

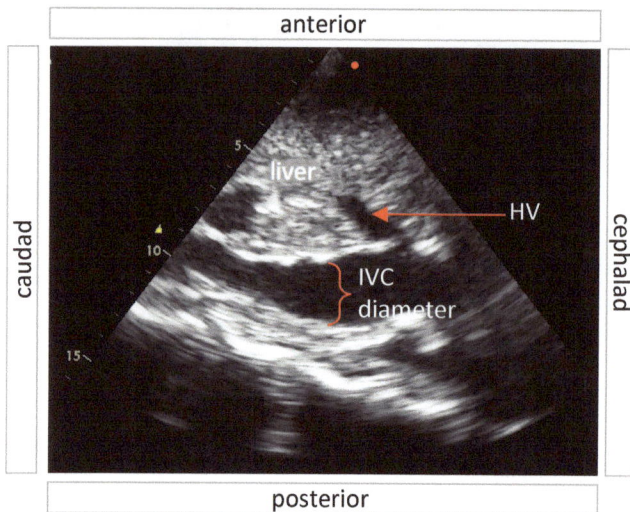

**Figure 5.8 Sagittal view of the inferior vena cava (IVC).**
The phased array probe is used here in the 'cardiac setting' hence the orientation marker is on the upper right hand side. HV: hepatic vein.

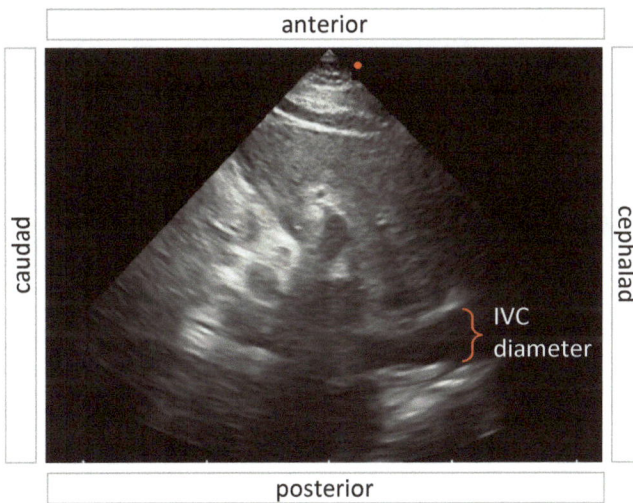

**Video 5.7 Significant respiratory variability of the inferior vena cava (IVC).**
Sagittal view of the IVC showing how the diameter of the IVC varies during respiration. In this example, there is complete collapse of the IVC during inspiration.
Video: bedsideultrasoundlevel1.com

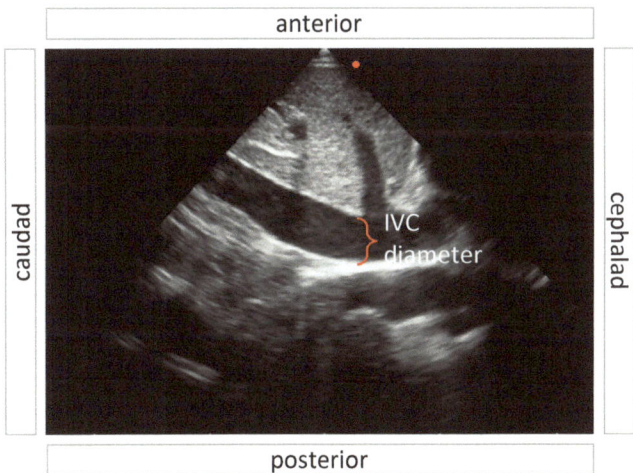

**Video 5.8 Minimal respiratory variability of the inferior vena cava (IVC).**
Sagittal view of the IVC showing a lack of IVC diameter respiratory variability.
Video: bedsideultrasoundlevel1.com

Studies have shown some correlation of a patient's volume status with both IVC diameter and its respiratory variability [24-27].

## Clinical relevance - Hypotensive patient

In a hypotensive patient:

- When hypovolemia is the cause of the hypotension, the IVC diameter is generally <15 mm and varies more than 50% with respiration

- The initial treatment usually involves an infusion of a volume expander (e.g. normal saline or Ringer's lactate). The effect of volume infusion can be evaluated with serial monitoring of the IVC diameter and respiratory variability. For example, adequate volume infusion given to a hypovolemic patient should increase the diameter and decrease the variability of the IVC [20]

- When either myocardial infarction, pulmonary embolism, or tamponade is the cause of the hypotension, the IVC diameter is generally >20 mm and varies less than 50% with respiration.

**Table 5.2 Summary table of the common causes of hypotension and their bedside ultrasound findings**

| Causes of hypotension | IVC | LV function |
|---|---|---|
| LV myocardial infarction | Large diameter and not variable | Moderate or severe LV dysfunction |
| Pulmonary embolism | Large diameter and not variable | Hyperdynamic LV function with increased RV:LV ratio |
| Tamponade | Large diameter and not variable | Hyperdynamic LV function and pericardial effusion (More advanced echocardiographic signs of tamponade are not covered in this introductory textbook.) |
| Hypovolemia | Small diameter and variable | Hyperdynamic LV function |
| Sepsis | Small diameter and variable. Late in sepsis, possibly large diameter and not variable | Commonly hyperdynamic LV function. Late in sepsis, possibly moderate or severe LV dysfunction |

## 5.7 Additional ultrasound assessments for hypotension

Additional focused bedside ultrasound examinations can help determine the cause of hypotension following the assessment of the LV function, RV:LV ratio, pericardium, and IVC.

For example:

- If tension pneumothorax is suspected, look for the absence of lung sliding (Chapter 4)

- If intraabdominal bleeding is suspected in trauma, look for free intraabdominal fluid (Chapter 6)

- If abdominal pain is present, look for an AAA (Chapter 7)

- If ectopic pregnancy is suspected, look for the absence of intra-uterine pregnancy (Chapter 11).

## 5.8 Troubleshooting tips

- When imaging the IVC, apply light pressure on the probe. Excessive pressure will collapse the IVC

- In a patient receiving positive pressure ventilation, the IVC diameter increases rather than decreases during inspiration

- To ensure that your probe is caudal to the liver, start your subxiphoid scan just above the umbilicus and move the probe slowly and superiorly on the abdomen. This is important because you require the liver to act as an acoustic window in order to obtain an acceptable subxiphoid view.

## 5.9 False-positives and false-negatives

---

**False-positives:**

- **Pericardial fat pad:** A pericardial fat pad can be confused for a pericardial effusion. Pericardial fat pads are hypoechoic (grey) and not anechoic (black). In addition, pericardial fat pads appear anteriorly, while pericardial effusions first present infero-posteriorly (due to gravity). Although it is possible to have a large pericardial effusion in both the posterior and anterior pericardium, pericardial effusions generally do not present in the anterior pericardium alone

- **Ascites and pleural effusion:** Ascites and pleural effusion can appear as an anechoic (black) structure next to the pericardium in the subxiphoid view of the heart and thus both ascites and pleural effusion can be false-positives for pericardial effusion.

---

## 5.10   CPoCUS documentation standards

The Canadian Point of Care Ultrasound Society (CPoCUS) recommends that POCUS exams be documented as follows:

- **Pericardial effusion (PCE):**

  o   Negative study:   PCE –

  o   Positive study:   PCE +

  o   Indeterminate:   PCE indeterminate

> ## Case closed:
>
> The 80 year old hypotensive man has a hyperdynamic LV, normal RV:LV ratio, no pericardial effusion, and a small variable IVC, suggesting hypovolemia. As volume expanders are administered, further ultrasound examination reveals a large ruptured abdominal aortic aneurysm. A vascular surgeon is urgently consulted.

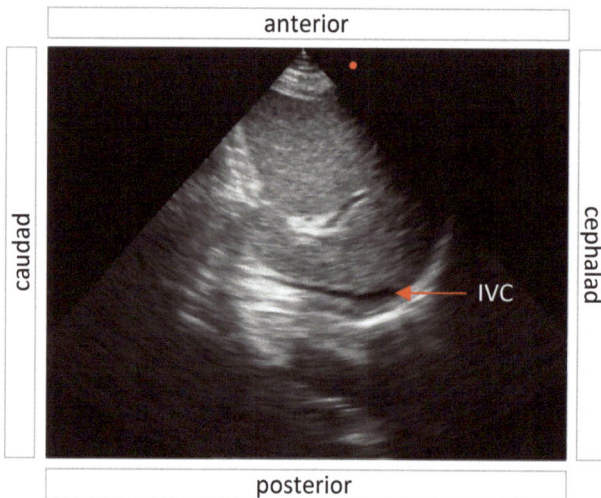

**Figure 5.9 Sagittal view of a small diameter inferior vena cava (IVC).**

# 6. Trauma

6.1  Probe choice

6.2  Patient position and scanning technique

6.3  The eFAST algorithm

6.4  Troubleshooting tips

6.5  False-positives and false-negatives

6.6  CPoCUS documentation standards

**Case scenario:**

A 25 year old woman is struck by a car and is brought to the emergency room by ambulance. She is conscious, and complains of abdominal and chest pain. Her blood pressure is 80/60 mmHg, and her heart rate is 120 beats/min. Her abdomen is tender without peritoneal signs.

**Impression:**

Hypotension in the setting of trauma. Rule out intraabdominal bleeding.

This chapter will introduce the use of bedside ultrasound in diagnosing intraabdominal/pelvic bleeding, hemopericardium, hemothorax, and pneumothorax in the setting of trauma.

## 6.1 Probe choice

Low frequency probes are used for this application. The curvilinear probe is most commonly used, however a phased array probe in the abdominal setting is also an appropriate choice.

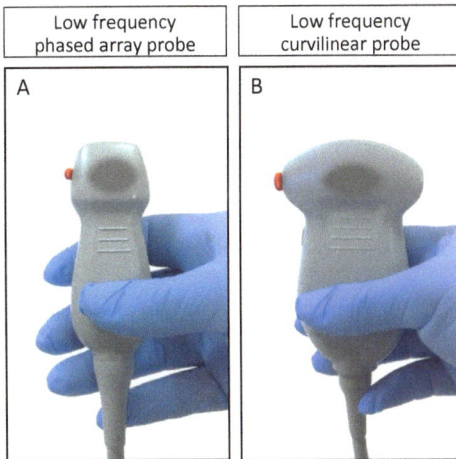

| Low frequency phased array probe | Low frequency curvilinear probe |
|---|---|
| A | B |

**Figure 6.1 Low frequency probes that can be used for assessing a trauma patient.**
**A.** A phased array probe.
**B.** A curvilinear probe.
Red circle denotes orientation marker.

## 6.2 Patient position and scanning technique

Patients are evaluated in the supine position.

## 6.3 The eFAST algorithm

Bedside ultrasound is useful in answering four questions in the setting of trauma [7]:

Question #1:   Does the patient have a hemoperitoneum?
             In the trauma patient, free intraabdominal or pelvic fluid
             is assumed to be blood until proven otherwise

Question #2:   Does the patient have a hemopericardium?
             In thoracic trauma, pericardial fluid is assumed to be
             blood until proven otherwise

Question #3:   Does the patient have a hemothorax?
             In the trauma patient, a pleural effusion is assumed to be
             a hemothorax until proven otherwise

Question #4:   Does the patient have a pneumothorax?

These questions can be answered using the **eFAST** algorithm.

| The eFAST acronym represents: | | |
|---|---|---|
| | e | = extended |
| | F | = Focused |
| | A | = Assessment |
| | S | = Sonography |
| | T | = Trauma |

The use of this approach in trauma patients is well supported by the medical literature [7, 28, 29]. This chapter provides a summary of the eFAST algorithm at the introductory level.

**Question #1: Does the patient have a hemoperitoneum?**

The presence of free intraabdominal or pelvic fluid can be detected by scanning the following three areas:

Area #1:  Morison's pouch

Area #2:  Spleno-renal space

Area #3:  Pelvis (pouch of Douglas in females and rectovesicular space in males).

**Area #1: Morison's pouch** is the potential space between the liver and the upper pole of the right kidney. This space is one of the first places in the abdomen in which free fluid accumulates. To locate free fluid in Morison's pouch, the probe is held on the right posterior axillary line at the level of the xiphoid in the coronal plane with the orientation marker pointing cephalad [7, 28-30].

The probe is moved cephalad to caudad in the coronal plane, or antero-posteriorly until Morison's pouch is visualized. Once Morison's pouch is identified, sweep slowly through the interface between the right kidney and the liver. Sweep until the kidney disappears from view both anteriorly and posteriorly. The interface includes any point of contact between the kidney and the liver. It is important to image the entire interface and the lower tip of the liver. The presence of free fluid in Morison's pouch will appear anechoic (black) on the ultrasound image.

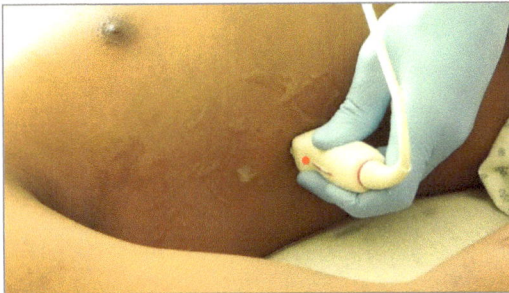

**Video 6.1 Scanning technique for imaging free fluid in Morison's pouch using a phased array probe.**
Video:
bedsideultrasoundlevel1.com

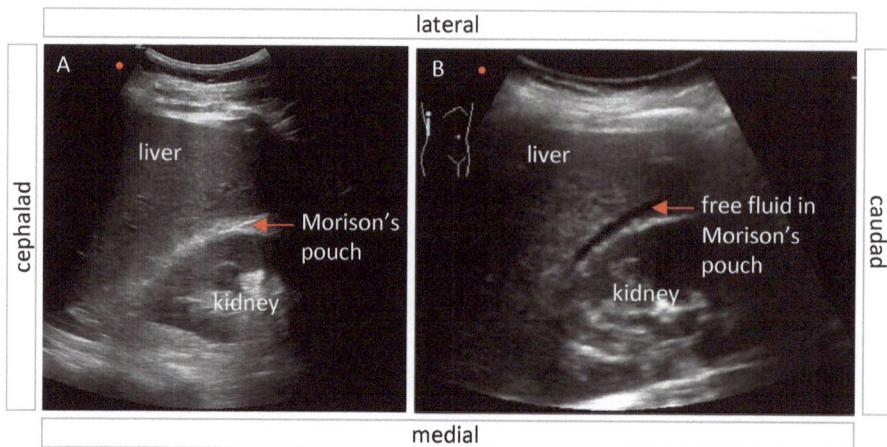

**Figure 6.2 Fluid in Morison's pouch revealed by a right posterolateral abdominal scan.**
**A.** The normal appearance of Morison's pouch. There is no anechoic (black) area between the liver and the right kidney.
**B.** Free fluid in Morison's pouch appears anechoic (black).

**Area #2: Spleno-renal space.** The spleno-renal space is the potential space between the spleen and the upper pole of the left kidney. To locate free fluid in the spleno-renal space, the probe is held on the left posterior axillary line at the level of the xiphoid in the coronal plane with the orientation marker pointing cephalad [7, 28, 29].

The probe is moved cephalad to caudad in the coronal plane, or antero-posteriorly until the examiner is able to visualize the spleno-renal interface. Sweep slowly through the interface between the left kidney and spleen. Sweep until the kidney disappears from view both anteriorly and posteriorly. The interface includes any point of contact between the kidney and the spleen. It is important to image the entire interface and the lower tip of the spleen. The presence of free fluid between the spleen and the left kidney will appear anechoic (black) on the ultrasound image.

In the left upper quadrant, the most dependent space is the sub-diaphragmatic area between the spleen and the diaphragm. Therefore, fluid may accumulate first in this area. It is essential that the interface between spleen and diaphragm be scanned from '6 to 9 o'clock' (see Figure 6.4).

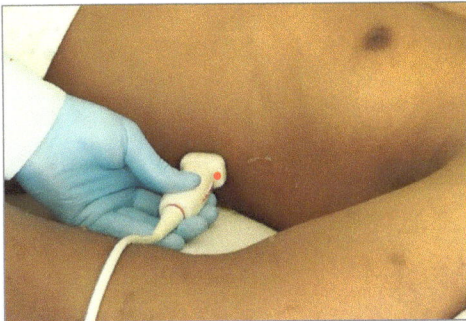

**Video 6.2 Scanning technique for imaging free fluid in the spleno-renal space using a phased array probe.**
Video:
bedsideultrasoundlevel1.com

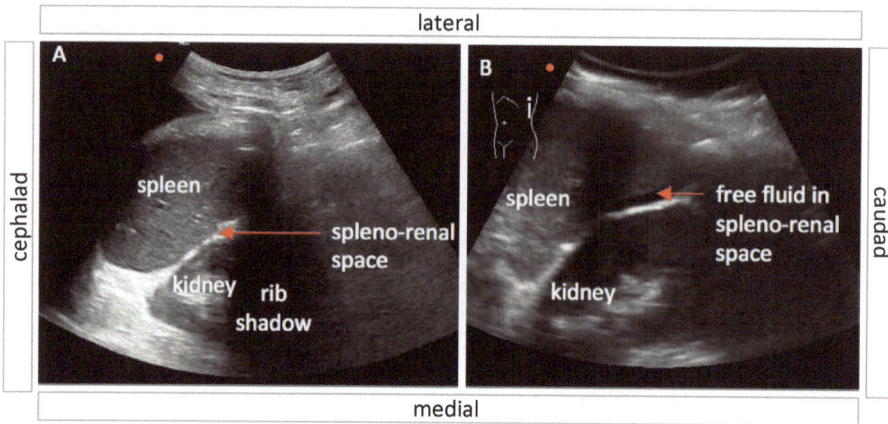

**Figure 6.3 Fluid in the spleno-renal space revealed by a left posterolateral abdominal scan.**
**A.** The normal appearance of the spleno-renal space.
**B.** Free fluid between the spleen and the left kidney appears anechoic (black).

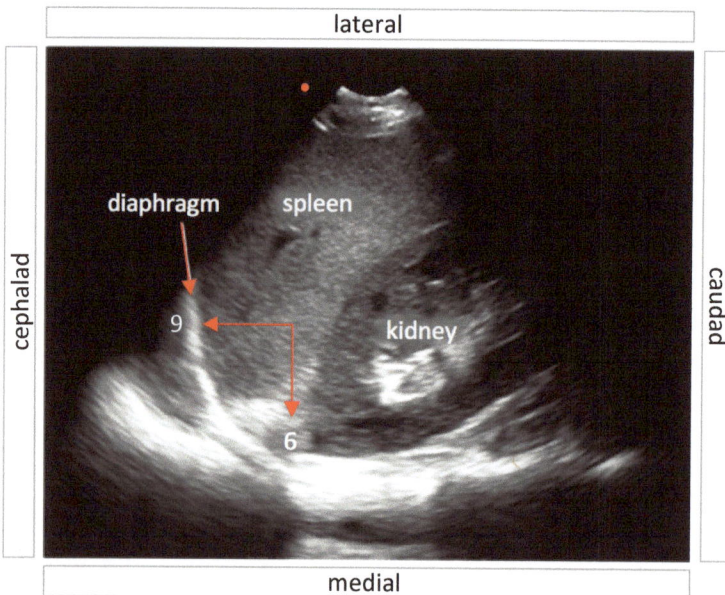

**Figure 6.4 The interface between spleen and diaphragm must be scanned from '6 to 9 o'clock' to look for sub-diaphragmatic fluid.**

**Area #3: Pelvis.** In females, free pelvic fluid collects between the bladder and the uterus, and in the **pouch of Douglas**. The pouch of Douglas is the potential space between the uterus and the rectum. Women of childbearing age may have a small amount of fluid in this space. In males, free pelvic fluid collects in the **rectovesicular space** between the bladder and the rectum [7, 28, 29].

To scan the pelvis in the transverse plane, place the probe just superior to the symphysis pubis with the orientation marker pointing to the patient's right. Tilt the probe so that it is aimed caudally. The urine filled bladder is appreciated as a large anechoic (black) structure in the near-field. In females, the uterus can be identified posterior to the bladder. The presence of free fluid will appear anechoic (black) posterior to the bladder or uterus in females and posterior to the bladder in males.

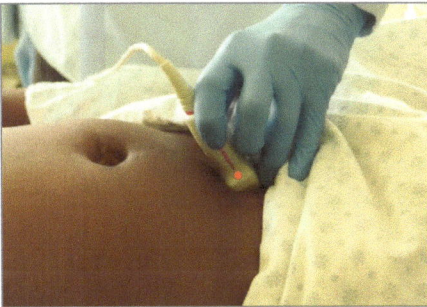

**Figure 6.5 Scanning technique for imaging the pelvis in the transverse plane using a phased array probe.**

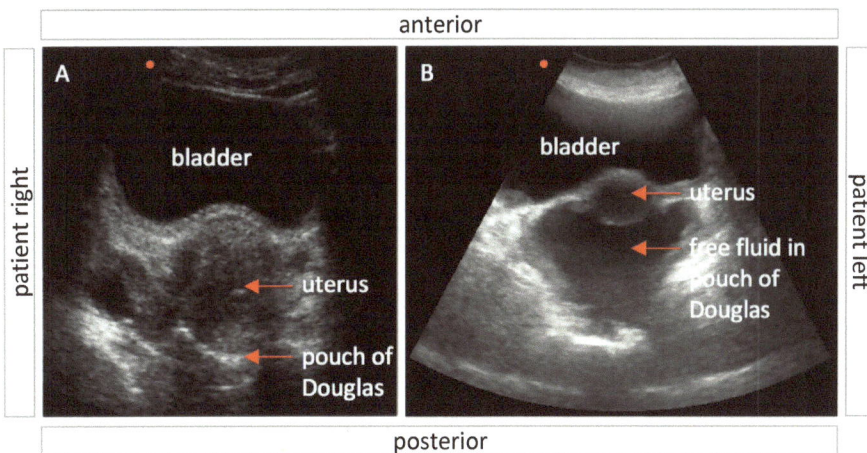

**Figure 6.6 The female pelvis in the transverse plane.**
**A.** The female pelvis without fluid in the pouch of Douglas.
**B.** The female pelvis with free fluid in the pouch of Douglas.

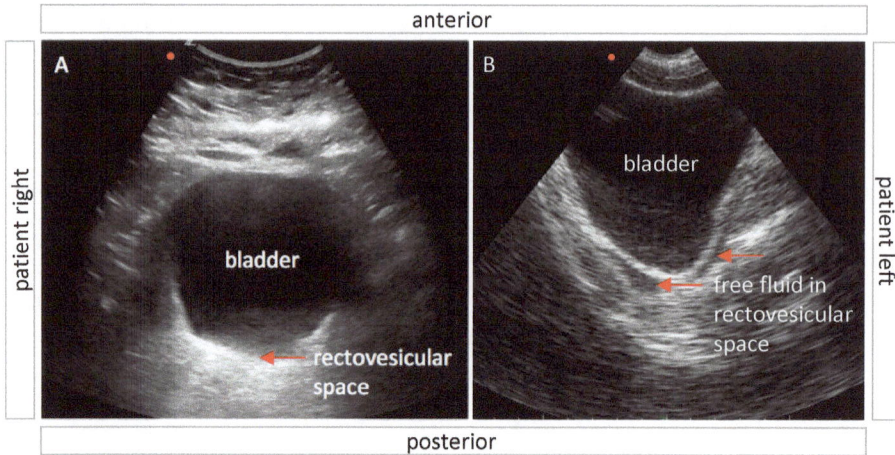

anterior

A

patient right

bladder

rectovesicular space

B

bladder

free fluid in rectovesicular space

patient left

posterior

**Figure 6.7 The male pelvis in the transverse plane.**
**A.** The male pelvis without fluid in the rectovesicular space.
**B.** The male pelvis with free fluid in the rectovesicular space.

To scan the pelvis in the sagittal plane, place the probe just superior to the symphysis pubis with the orientation marker pointing cephalad. Point the probe caudally.

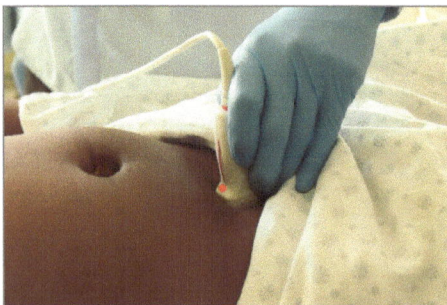

**Figure 6.8 Scanning technique for imaging the pelvis in the sagittal plane using a phased array probe.**

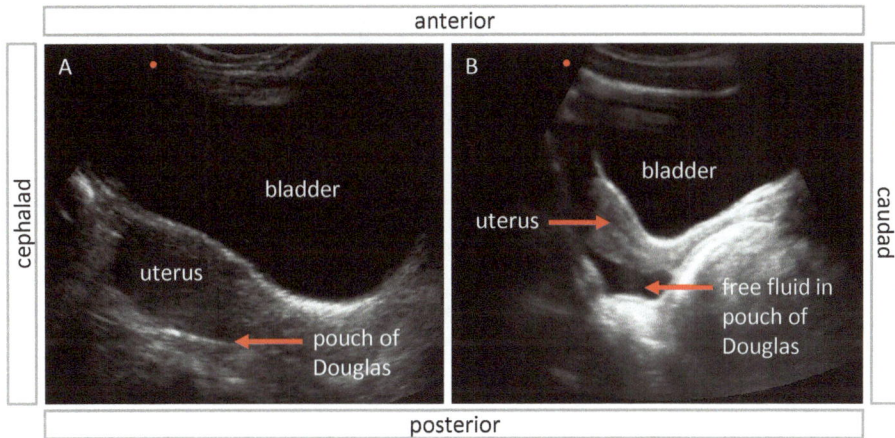

**Figure 6.9 The female pelvis in the sagittal plane.**
**A.** The female pelvis in sagittal plane without fluid in the pouch of Douglas.
**B.** The female pelvis in sagittal plane with free fluid in the pouch of Douglas.

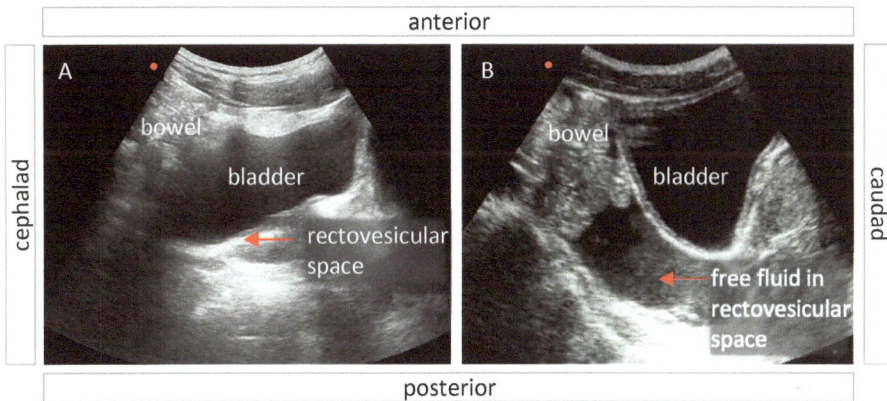

**Figure 6.10 The male pelvis in the sagittal plane.**
**A.** The male pelvis in sagittal plane without fluid in the rectovesicular space.
**B.** The male pelvis in sagittal plane with free fluid in the rectovesicular space.

**Summary:** If a trauma patient has free fluid in one of the three areas (Morison's pouch, spleno-renal space, pelvis), then the clinician suspects intraabdominal/pelvic bleeding.

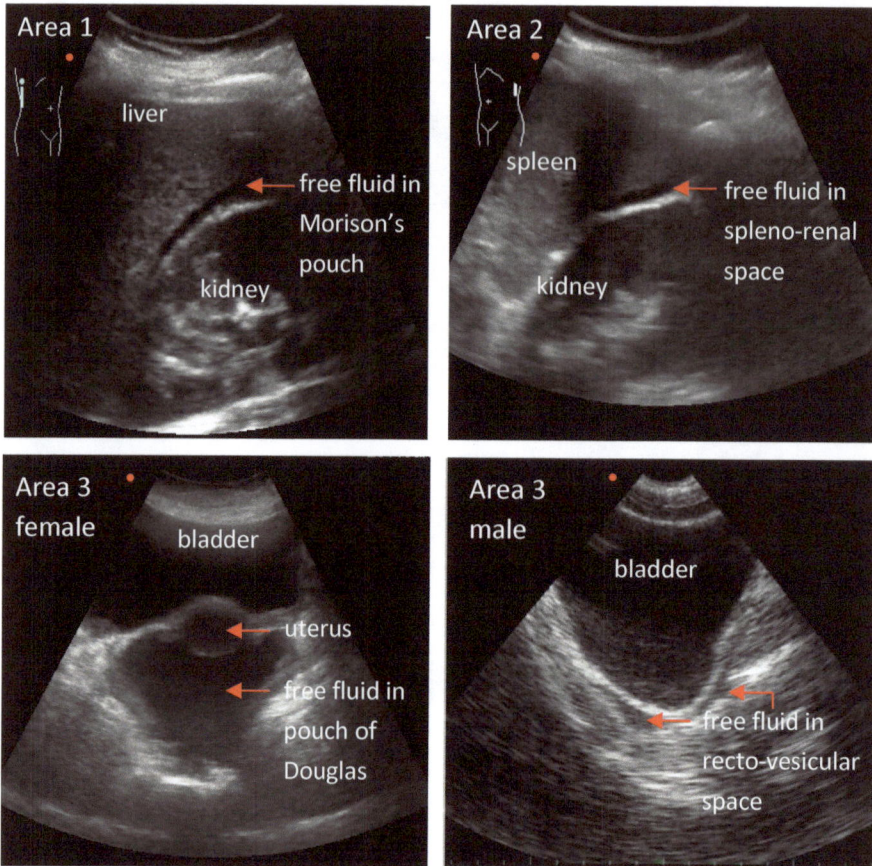

Figure 6.11 Free fluid in one of the three areas (Morison's pouch, spleno-renal space, pelvis) suggests intraabdominal/pelvic bleeding in the trauma patient.

## Question #2: Does the patient have a hemopericardium?

In the trauma patient, pericardial fluid is assumed to be blood until proven otherwise.

To look for pericardial fluid, image the heart using the subxiphoid view (for review see Section 5.5).

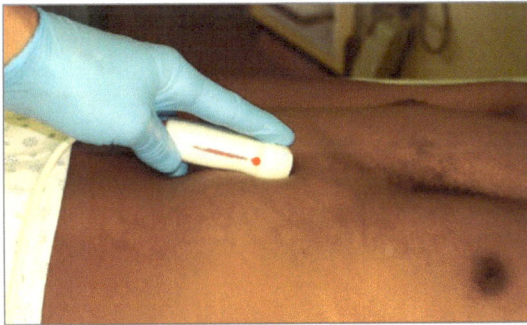

**Figure 6.12 Scanning technique for imaging pericardial fluid in the subxiphoid view.**
The orientation marker on the phased array probe in the cardiac setting points to patient's left. When using a curvilinear probe in the abdominal setting, the orientation marker points to patient's right.

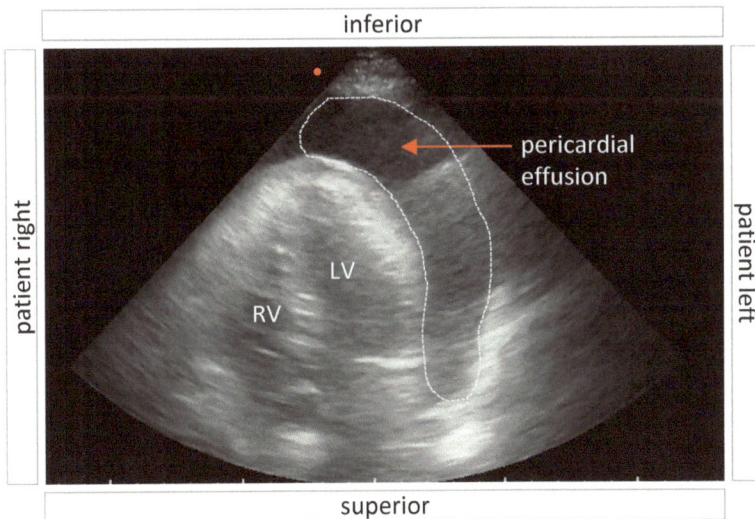

**Figure 6.13 A pericardial effusion seen in the subxiphoid view.**
The pericardial effusion appears as an anechoic (black) area around the heart.
RV: right ventricle, LV: left ventricle.

**Question #3: Does the patient have a hemothorax?**

In the trauma patient, a pleural effusion is assumed to be a hemothorax until proven otherwise.

Pleural effusions develop posteriorly in a supine patient. With the patient supine or semi-seated in bed, place the probe in the posterior axillary line in the coronal plane with the probe marker pointing cephalad (see also Section 4.7). A pleural effusion appears as an anechoic (black) area cephalad to the diaphragm. Atelectatic lung can sometimes be appreciated floating in the effusion. In addition, the presence of a **spine sign** suggests a pleural effusion (see Section 4.7).

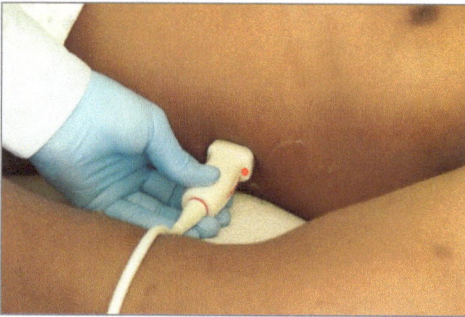

**Figure 6.14 Scanning technique for imaging a hemothorax in the left posterolateral chest using a phased array probe.**

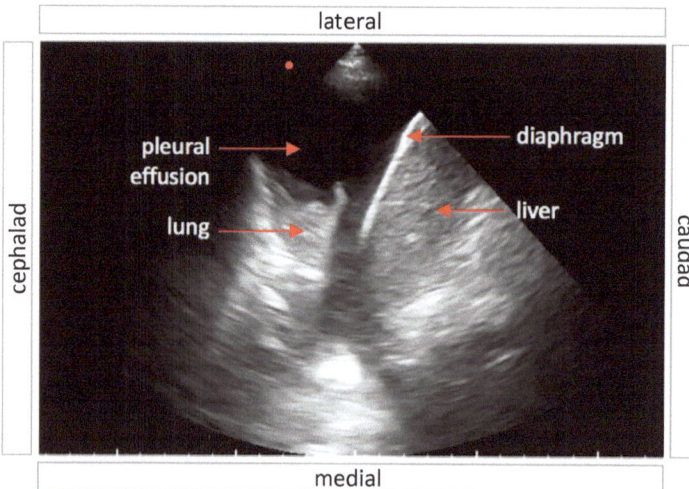

**Figure 6.15 A pleural effusion seen in a left posterolateral chest scan.**
The pleural effusion appears as an anechoic (black) area above the diaphragm.

**Question #4: Does the patient have a pneumothorax?**

A pneumothorax is common in the setting of major trauma. A pneumothorax is the accumulation of air between the parietal and visceral pleurae.

In a supine patient, a pneumothorax accumulates anteriorly and thus an anterior chest scan is essential. In the setting of trauma:

- The presence of lung sliding, 'B' lines, or a lung pulse on an anterior chest exam of a supine patient rules out a pneumothorax (Chapter 4)

- The absence of lung sliding suggests but is not conclusive for a pneumothorax (Chapter 4).

The identification of a pneumothorax on an ultrasound image is explained in detail in Section 4.3 [5-7, 31].

## 6.4 Troubleshooting tips

- If the image generated during an eFAST exam is suboptimal, the examination is indeterminate. Do not make clinical decisions based on suboptimal images

- If the subxiphoid view of the heart is unavailable due to abdominal pain, use other ultrasound views of the heart

- Ultrasound examination of the pelvis is easier when the bladder is full.

## 6.5 False-positives and false-negatives

**False-positives:** There are several structures that appear anechoic (black) on ultrasound, and can mimic hemoperitoneum in the setting of trauma. These include:

- Fluid within the bowel lumen
- Ascites (e.g. patient with cirrhosis who is involved in trauma)
- Peritoneal dialysate (patient on peritoneal dialysis who is involved in trauma)
- The prostate in a male
- Physiologic pelvic fluid in a female.

**False-negatives:** **There are two important clinical scenarios in which even a skillful bedside ultrasound independent practitioner can miss a hemoperitoneum:**

- **First scenario:** When the trauma patient presents hours after an injury. In delayed presentations, the hemoperitoneum coagulates to form a hematoma. The blood gradually transforms from anechoic (black), to hypoechoic (grey) and eventually to hyperechoic (white) on ultrasound. The ultrasonographer may fail to recognize a hemoperitoneum because the blood is no longer black in color on ultrasound

- **Second scenario:** In trauma patients who have had many previous abdominal surgeries. Intra-abdominal adhesions caused by previous surgeries can cause loculations of fluid in the setting of hemoperitoneum. Blood may not accumulate in the usual places (right and left upper quadrants, pelvis).

## 6.6 CPoCUS documentation standards

The Canadian Point of Care Ultrasound Society (CPoCUS) recommends that POCUS exams be documented as follows:

- **Free fluid (FF):**

  o   Negative study:    FF –

  o   Positive study:    FF +

  o   Indeterminate:    FF indeterminate

**Case closed:**

The 25 year old trauma patient is found to have free fluid in Morison's pouch and the spleno-renal space on ultrasound examination. She is presumed to have intra-abdominal bleeding secondary to trauma. As volume expanders are administered, a trauma surgeon is consulted.

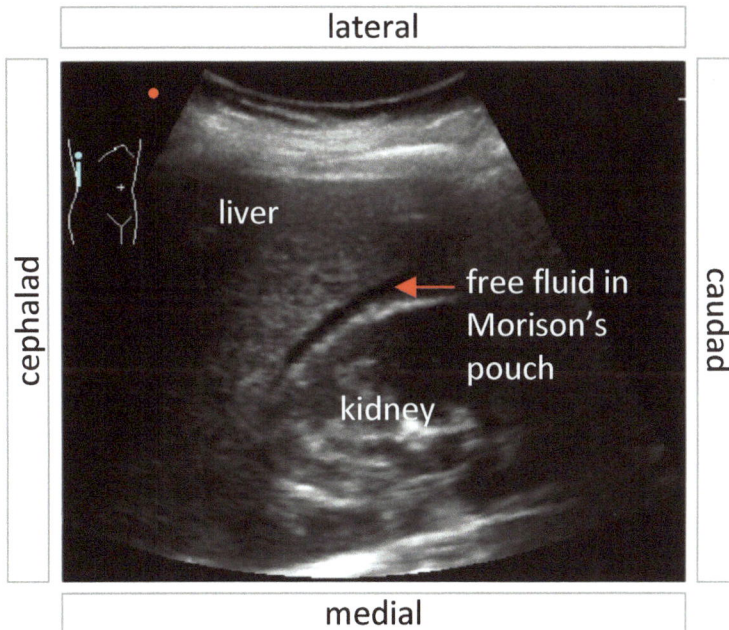

**Figure 6.16 Free fluid in Morison's pouch.**

# 7. ABDOMINAL AORTIC ANEURYSM (AAA)

7.1  Probe choice

7.2  Patient position and scanning technique

7.3  Using bedside ultrasound to identify an AAA

7.4  Troubleshooting tips

7.5  False-positives and false-negatives

7.6  CPoCUS documentation standards

> **Case scenario:**
>
> A 70 year old man presents himself to the clinic complaining of abdominal pain that is radiating to his back. His only medication is an ACE inhibitor for hypertension. His heart rate is 100 beats per minute, his blood pressure is 90/40 mmHg, and he appears to be in distress. Due to his obesity, it is difficult to palpate deep abdominal structures on a physical exam.
>
> **Impression:**
>
> Abdominal pain not yet determined, rule out an abdominal aortic aneurysm.

An **abdominal aortic aneurysm (AAA)** is a localized dilation of the abdominal aorta. This chapter will review the technique for imaging the abdominal aorta with bedside ultrasound and illustrate how to recognize an AAA.

## 7.1 Probe choice

To image the abdominal aorta, use a low frequency probe such as a phased array probe (in the abdominal setting) or a curvilinear probe. Low frequency probes provide the depth penetration needed to image deep structures like the abdominal aorta.

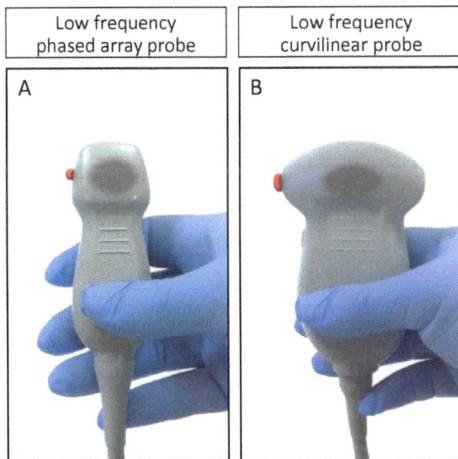

**Figure 7.1 Low frequency probes that can be used to assess a patient with a suspected abdominal aortic aneurysm (AAA).**
**A.** A phased array probe.
**B.** A curvilinear probe.
Red circle denotes orientation marker.

## 7.2 Patient position and scanning technique

The patient should be in the supine position, with the knees slightly bent to relax the abdominal musculature. Start in the epigastric area immediately caudal to the xiphoid process with the probe held in the transverse plane. The orientation marker should point to the patient's right. Identify the abdominal aorta first and then scan in the transverse plane every centimeter down to the bifurcation of the aorta into the iliac arteries [32, 33].

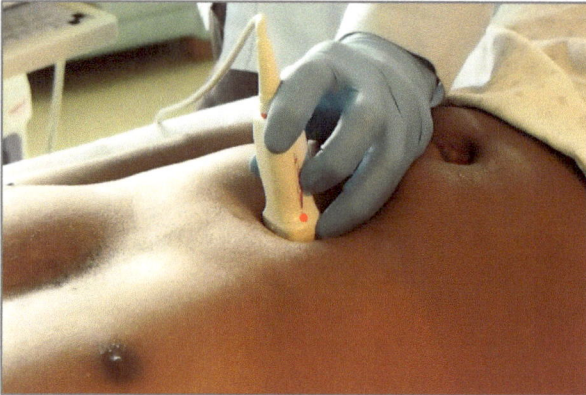

**Video 7.1 Scanning technique for imaging the abdominal aorta in the transverse plane.**
Video: bedsideultrasoundlevel1.com

The internal landmark used to identify the aorta on the ultrasound image is the **vertebral body.** The anterior aspect of the vertebral body appears as a hyperechoic (white) structure. The vertebral body casts a shadow deep to its hyperechoic surface because ultrasound cannot penetrate bone. The abdominal aorta appears as a round anechoic (black) structure, immediately anterior and usually to the screen-right of the vertebral body on the ultrasound monitor.

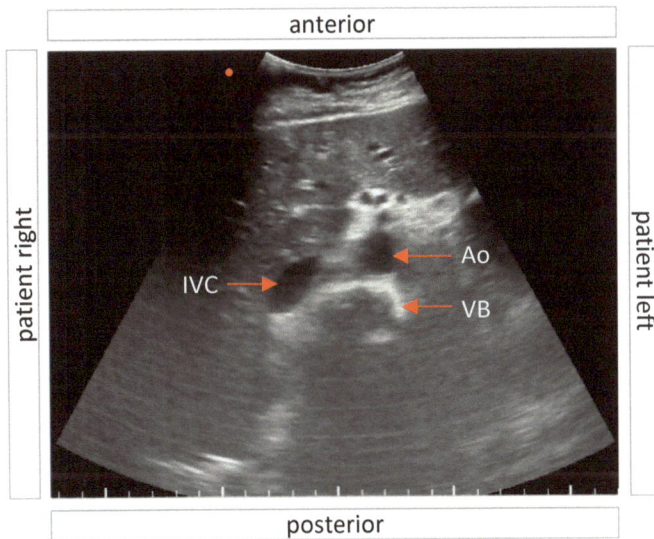

**Figure 7.2 The abdominal aorta in the transverse plane.**
The aorta (Ao) is anterior and to the right of the vertebral body (VB). The inferior vena cava (IVC) is also anterior but to the left of the vertebral body.

**Table 7.1 Characteristics of the ultrasound image used to differentiate the abdominal aorta from the inferior vena cava (IVC)**

| Characteristics | Abdominal aorta | IVC |
| --- | --- | --- |
| Shape | Round | Tear-shaped |
| Walls | Thick | Thin |
| Respiratory variability in diameter | No | Yes |
| Position relative to vertebral body | Anterior, usually screen-right | Anterior, screen-left |
| Compressibility | Non-compressible | Compressible |

A determinate transverse scan is sufficient when scanning for an AAA and thus imaging the aorta in the sagittal plane is not obligatory. If a sagittal scan is requested, locate the aorta in the transverse plane, then rotate the probe clockwise 90°. The aorta is now imaged in the sagittal plane. The proximal aorta will be on screen-left and the distal aorta on screen-right.

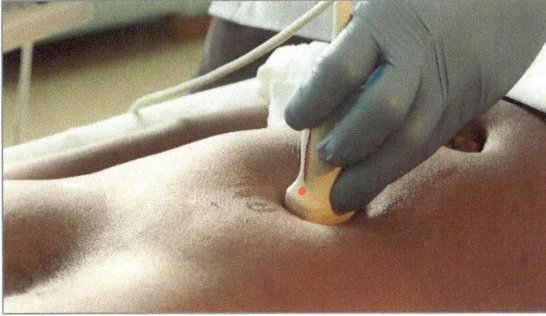

**Video 7.2 Scanning technique for imaging the abdominal aorta in the sagittal plane with a phased array probe.**
Video:
bedsideultrasoundlevel1.com

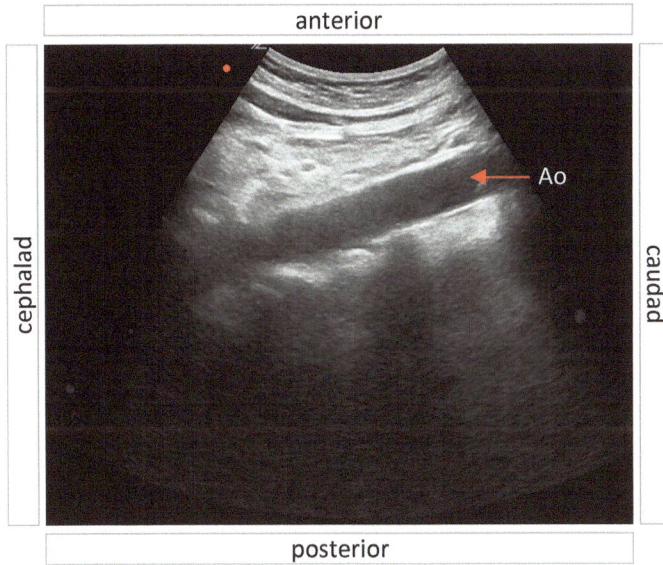

**Figure 7.3 The abdominal aorta in the sagittal plane.**
Ao: Aorta.

## 7.3 Using bedside ultrasound to identify an AAA

Bedside ultrasound is accurate in diagnosing an AAA [34] yet insensitive in identifying the presence of retroperitoneal blood associated with a ruptured AAA [35]. Therefore, the objective of bedside ultrasound is to identify the presence or absence of an AAA rather than determine whether the AAA is ruptured or not. Whether the AAA is ruptured or not will be determined with other imaging modalities (e.g. CT abdomen).

**Clinical relevance - Abdominal aortic aneurysm**

An AAA is present when the diameter of the aorta is greater than 3 cm. The diameter of the aorta should be measured from outer wall to outer wall at the point of maximum diameter. Take the measurement in the orientation in which the diameter is maximum. The orientation could be antero-posterior or lateral to lateral wall.

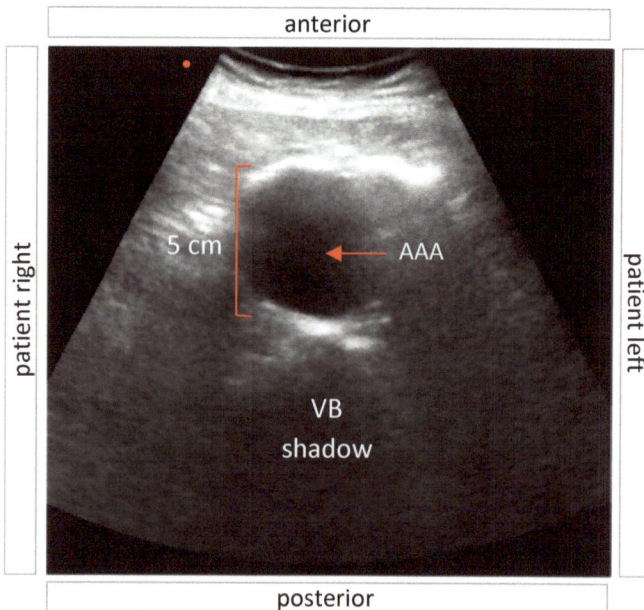

**Figure 7.4 An abdominal aortic aneurysm (AAA) in the transverse plane.**
The diameter of the aorta is greater than 3 cm from outer wall to outer wall. VB: vertebral body.

An intraluminal clot within an AAA may falsely suggest a normal aortic diameter. This is because the edge of the clot may be mistaken for the aortic wall.

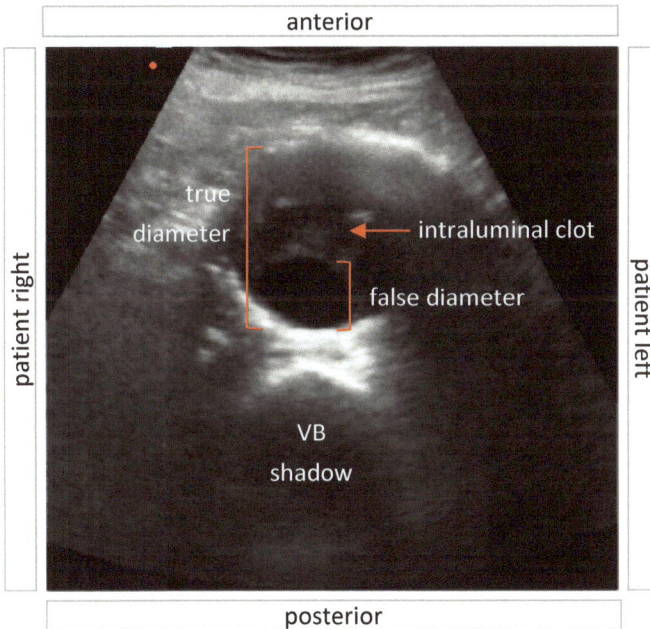

**Figure 7.5 An abdominal aortic aneurysm (AAA) with intraluminal clot.**
The true diameter of the AAA is 7 cm. VB: vertebral body.

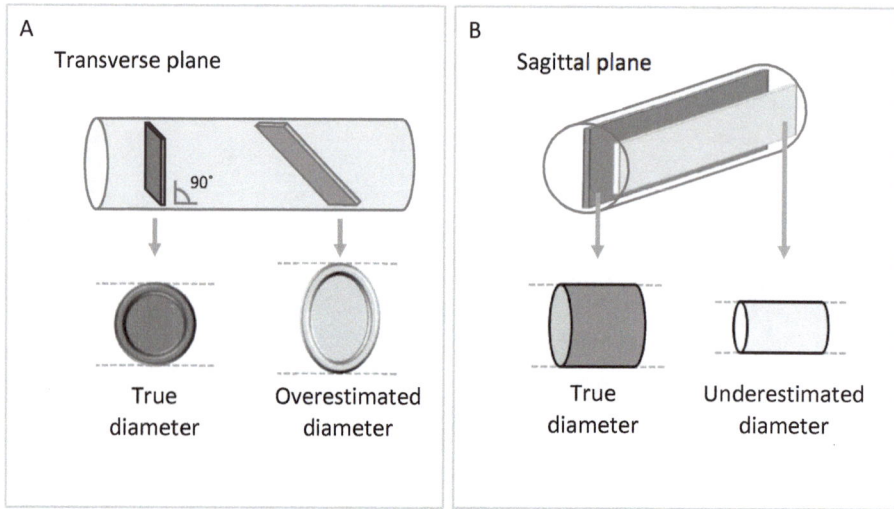

**Figure 7.6 Estimating the true aortic diameter in the transverse and sagittal plane.**
**A.** Estimating the aortic diameter in the transverse plane must be performed with the plane of view perpendicular to the vessel.
**B.** Estimating the aortic diameter in the sagittal plane must be performed with the plane of view at the center of the vessel.

## 7.4 Troubleshooting tips

- Bowel gas sometimes obscures the image of the abdominal aorta. To move the bowel out of the way, apply gentle pressure on the abdomen with the probe and wait for 30 seconds as peristalsis moves the bowel out of the way. Asking the patient to take a large breath may also move the bowel out of the way

- In obese patients, the abdominal aorta may be difficult to image. Image generation can be facilitated by:

  o Starting the scan with the depth setting at maximum

  o Placing patients in the left or right lateral decubitus position. This causes the abdominal skin and adipose to fall out of the way allowing better access to the aorta

  o Approaching the scan to the left of midline and rocking the probe medially

  o Lowering the frequency of the probe to increase penetration of the ultrasound beam.

- Gas in the umbilicus can cast a shadow and obscure the aorta at the level of its bifurcation. This can be avoided by filling the umbilicus with gel or approaching the scan from left of midline at the level of the umbilicus.

## 7.5 False-positives and false-negatives

**False-positives:**

- **Overestimation of aorta diameter:** The diameter of the aorta may seem to be greater than 3 cm and thus falsely suggest an AAA in a transverse image in which the probe is not perpendicular to the aorta (see Figure 7.6)

- **Lymphadenopathy:** A patient with lymphadenopathy may have large para-aortic lymph nodes that appear hypoechoic and circular, and falsely mimic an AAA.

## 7.6 CPoCUS documentation standards

The Canadian Point of Care Ultrasound Society (CPoCUS) recommends that POCUS exams be documented as follows:

- **Abdominal aortic aneurysm (AAA):**
  - Diameter ≤ 3 cm:  AAA < 3 cm
  - Diameter > 3 cm:  AAA __ cm
  - Indeterminate:    AAA indeterminate

**Case closed:**

The 70 year old man is found to have a large 5 cm AAA on ultrasound examination. The AAA was visualized upon placing the patient in the right lateral decubitus position. A vascular surgeon is urgently consulted.

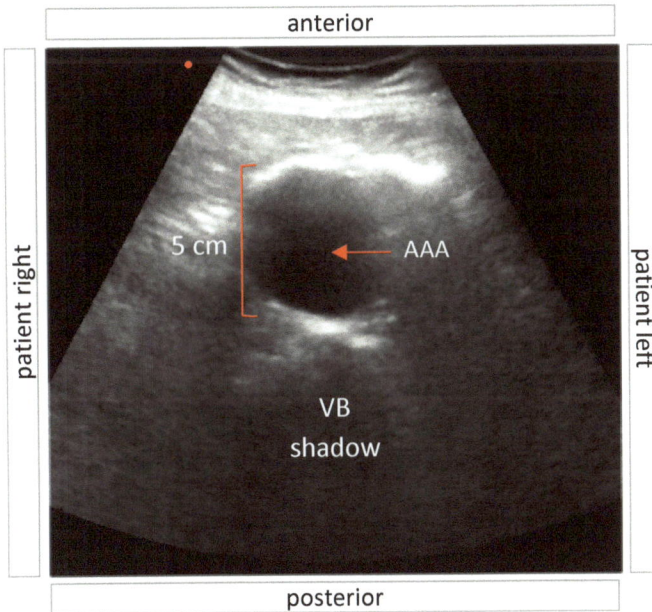

**Figure 7.7 An abdominal aortic aneurysm (AAA) in the transverse plane.**
VB: vertebral body.

# 8. CHOLECYSTITIS

8.1  Probe choice

8.2  Patient position and scanning technique

8.3  Ultrasound appearance of the gallbladder

8.4  Troubleshooting tips

8.5  False-positives and false-negatives

8.6  CPoCUS documentation standards

Case scenario:

A 60 year old obese man with no significant past medical history presents himself to the clinic with postprandial abdominal pain. Examination reveals a man with a fever of 38.5°C, otherwise normal vital signs, and right upper quadrant tenderness on palpation.

Impression:

Abdominal pain, must rule out cholecystitis.

**Cholecystitis** is an inflammation of the gallbladder often caused by the obstruction of the cystic duct by gallstones. This chapter will review the technique for imaging the gallbladder with bedside ultrasound and illustrate the basic ultrasonographic signs of cholecystitis.

## 8.1 Probe choice

To image the gallbladder, use a low frequency probe such as a phased array probe (in the abdominal setting) or a curvilinear probe. Low frequency probes provide the depth penetration necessary to image deep structures like the gallbladder.

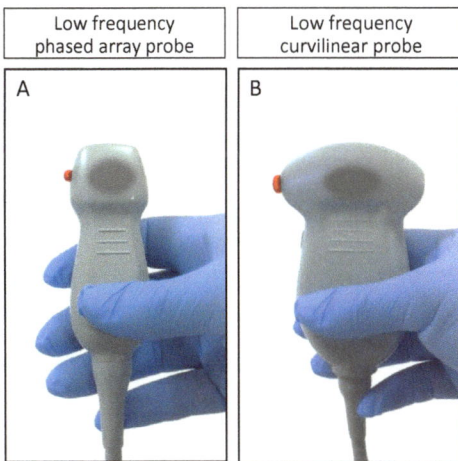

**Figure 8.1 Low frequency probes that can be used to assess a patient with suspected cholecystitis.**
**A.** A phased array probe.
**B.** A curvilinear probe.
Red circle denotes orientation marker.

## 8.2 Patient position and scanning technique

There are four basic scanning techniques to image the gallbladder in a supine patient:

Scanning technique #1:  The subcostal sweep

Scanning technique #2:  Left lateral decubitus

Scanning technique #3:  The X-7 approach

Scanning technique #4:  The posterolateral approach.

**Scanning technique #1: The subcostal sweep**

The patient lies in the supine position with knees slightly bent in order to relax the abdominal muscles. The probe is held in the sagittal plane with the orientation marker pointing cephalad. Place the probe below the costal margin in the epigastric area and sweep along the right costal margin laterally.

In general, the gallbladder will come into view in the right subcostal area at the mid-clavicular line. Since the gallbladder is generally under the ribs, the probe must be rocked so that it is pointing slightly cephalad.

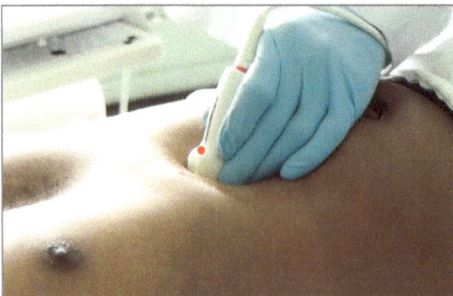

**Video 8.1 Scanning technique #1: The subcostal sweep for imaging the gallbladder.**
The gallbladder is generally found in the mid-clavicular line. Video: bedsideultrasoundlevel1.com

## Scanning technique #2: Left lateral decubitus

Ask the patient to lie on their left side (left lateral decubitus) and repeat the subcostal sweep. This maneuver can help move the gallbladder from beneath the ribs and allows the bowel overlying the gallbladder to fall away toward the bed. This improves the ability to identify the gallbladder.

## Scanning technique #3: The X-7 approach

The 'X' refers to the xiphoid region. The probe is placed 7 cm lateral and to the right of the xiphoid. The probe is held in the transverse plane with the orientation marker pointing towards the patient's right. The probe angle must be adjusted such that the ultrasound beam penetrates the intercostal space and avoids the ribs. The gallbladder will often be found at this location.

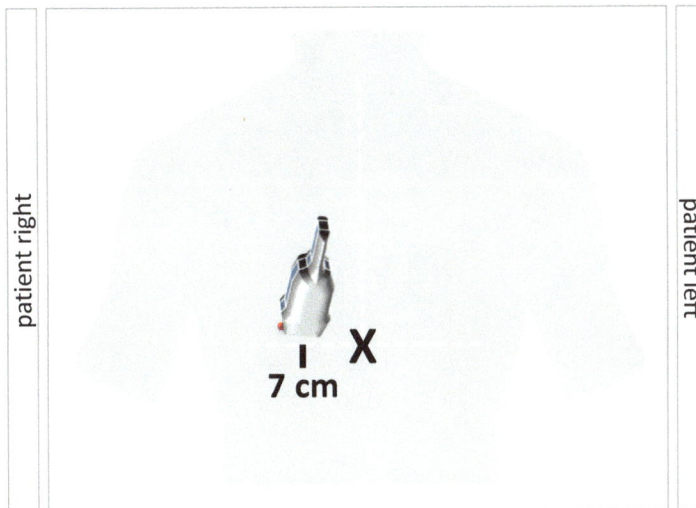

**Figure 8.2 Scanning technique #3: The X-7 technique for imaging the gallbladder.**
The probe is placed 7 cm laterally and to the right of the xiphoid (**X**).

## Scanning technique #4: The posterolateral approach

The probe is placed over the right posterolateral flank with the orientation marker pointing cephalad. Once Morison's pouch has been identified (the potential space between the liver and the upper pole of the right kidney; Section 6.3), the probe is moved anteriorly until the gallbladder comes into view.

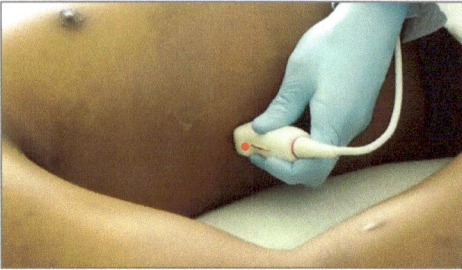

**Video 8.2 Scanning technique #4: The posterolateral approach for imaging the gallbladder.**
Video: bedsideultrasoundlevel1.com

## 8.3 Ultrasound appearance of the gallbladder

A normal gallbladder appears as an anechoic (black) structure with thin hyperechoic (white) walls. The gallbladder is surrounded by the hypoechoic (grey) appearing liver. Depending on its position, you may first see the gallbladder in the short or longitudinal orientation. A useful landmark to identify the gallbladder in the longitudinal orientation is the **exclamation point sign**. The exclamation point sign is formed by the pear-shaped gallbladder in longitudinal orientation and the right portal vein in transverse orientation.

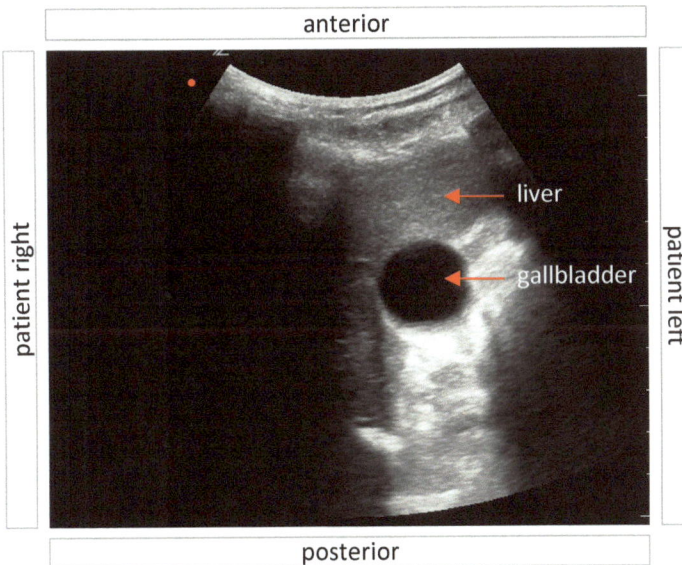

Figure 8.3 The gallbladder imaged in the short orientation.

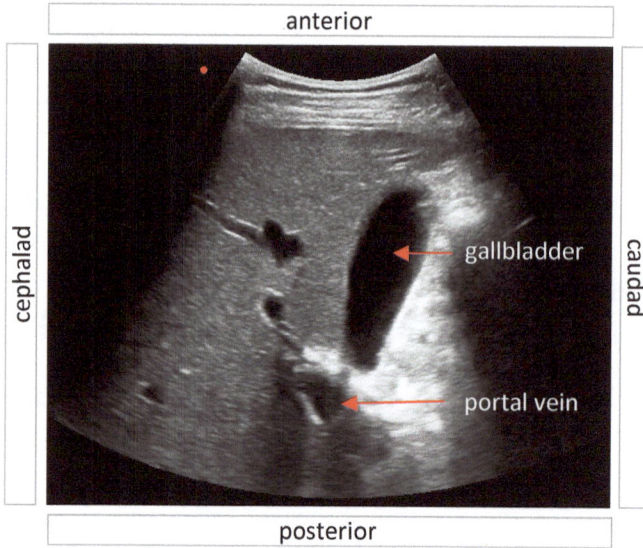

**Figure 8.4 The exclamation point sign: gallbladder imaged in the longitudinal orientation.**

The exclamation point sign is formed by the gallbladder in longitudinal orientation and the portal vein in transverse orientation.

It is important to scan through the gallbladder in **both the short and the longitudinal orientation**. First find the gallbladder in the longitudinal orientation and sweep through it from side-to-side. Then rotate the probe counterclockwise and sweep through the gallbladder from the fundus to the neck in the short orientation.

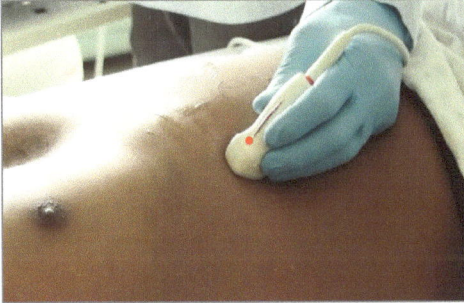

**Video 8.3 Scanning technique for imaging the gallbladder in the longitudinal and short orientation using a phased array probe.**
Video: bedsideultrasoundlevel1.com

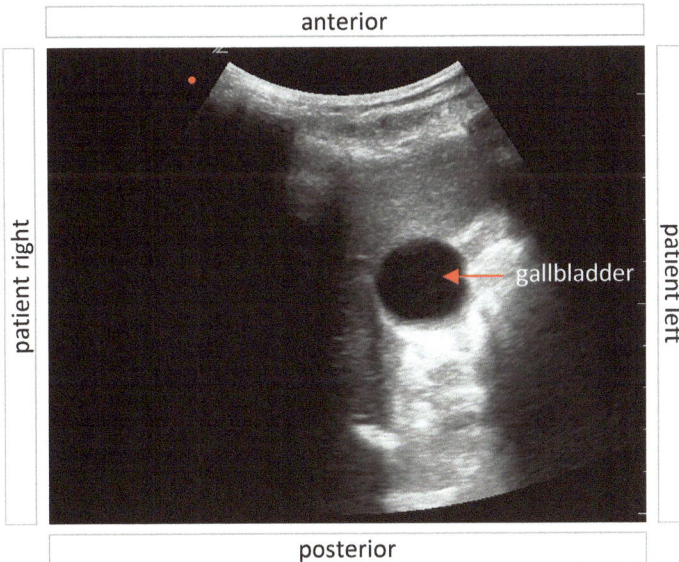

**Video 8.4 The gallbladder being imaged in the short orientation from the fundus to the neck.**
Video: bedsideultrasoundlevel1.com

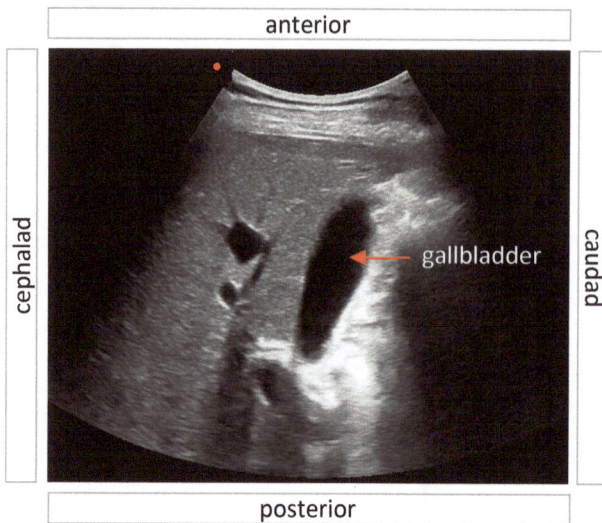

**Video 8.5 The gallbladder being imaged in the longitudinal orientation from side-to-side.**
Video: bedsideultrasoundlevel1.com

## Clinical relevance - Cholecystitis

Cholecystitis is often caused by the obstruction of the cystic duct by gallstones. Five important ultrasonographic signs to look for in diagnosing cholecystitis are:

Cholecystitis sign #1:  Gallstones

Cholecystitis sign #2:  Sonographic Murphy sign

Cholecystitis sign #3:  Thickening of anterior gallbladder wall

Cholecystitis sign #4:  Pericholecystic fluid

Cholecystitis sign #5:  Gallbladder distension.

**Cholecystitis sign #1. Gallstones**

Stones within the gallbladder are referred to as either **cholelithiasis** or **gallstones**. Gallstones appear hyperechoic (white) and cast a shadow into the far-field of the ultrasound image. The presence of a shadow differentiates gallstones from structures that do not cast a shadow such as gallbladder polyps, tumors, or thickened bile (sludge).

The false-positives for gallstone shadows are the refraction (edge) artifact and bowel gas (see Section 8.6). A refraction artifact can be created by the gallbladder and can resemble a gallstone shadow (see Section 3.6). Shadows cast from bowel are generally diffuse and hypoechoic (grey) and are referred to as 'dirty' shadows. Gallstone shadows are well delineated and anechoic (black) and referred to as 'clean' shadows.

The false-negatives for gallstone shadows are small gallstones less than 4 mm that may not cast a shadow. In this situation, a shadow can sometimes be appreciated by increasing the frequency of the ultrasound.

Most gallstones are mobile and lie on the dependent side of the gallbladder. Therefore, this characteristic can be useful in identifying a gallstone - if the patient changes position, the gallstone will move and settle to the dependent side of the gallbladder. However, there are three exceptions to this rule:

1.  Cholesterol gallstones float and so do not settle to the dependent side of the gallbladder

2.  Gallstones that are impacted in the neck of the gallbladder will not move as the patient changes position

3.  'WES' sign occurs when the gallbladder lumen is completely full of gallstones. On ultrasound the **WES** sign is caused by the **W**all of the gallbladder in the near-field, the gallbladder lumen full of **E**chogenic stones and then a **S**hadow cast by the stones into the far-field.

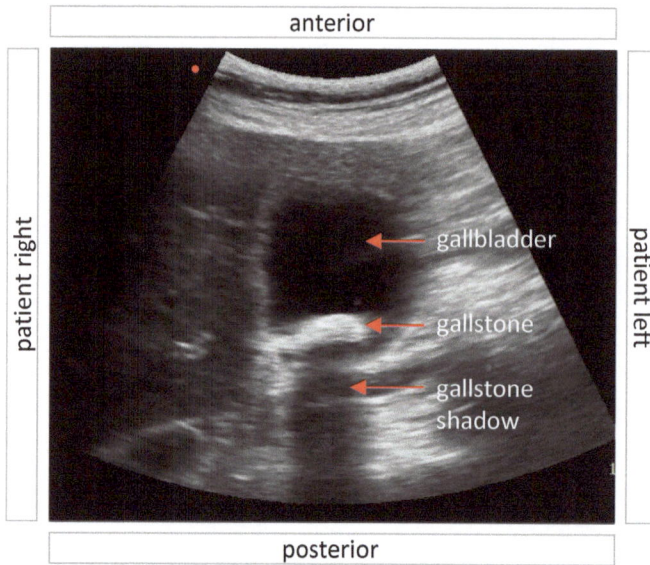

**Figure 8.5 The gallbladder in transverse orientation showing a gallstone.**
Gallstones appear as hyperechoic (white) structures within the gallbladder lumen. They cast a dark shadow into the far-field of the ultrasound screen.

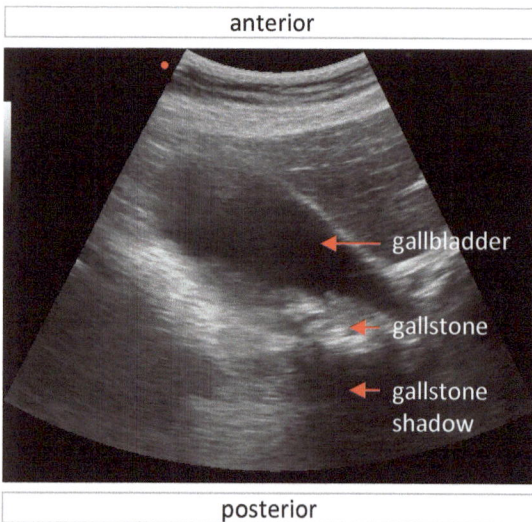

**Figure 8.6 The gallbladder in the longitudinal orientation showing gallstones at the neck of the gallbladder.**
The gallstones cast a shadow.

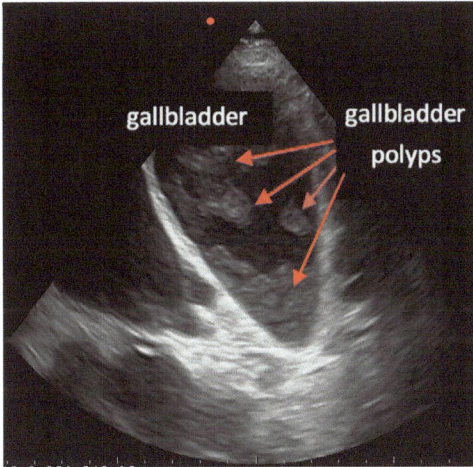

**Figure 8.7 The gallbladder in the longitudinal orientation showing multiple gallbladder polyps.**
Gallbladder polyps do not cast shadows.

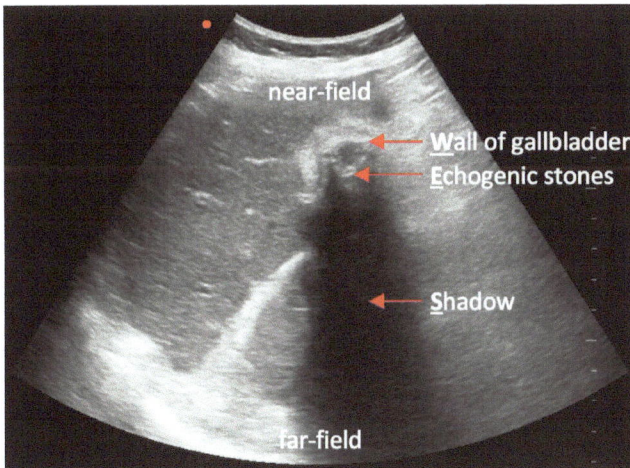

**Figure 8.8 WES sign.**
Note that the gallbladder lumen is full of echogenic stones that cast a shadow into the far-field.

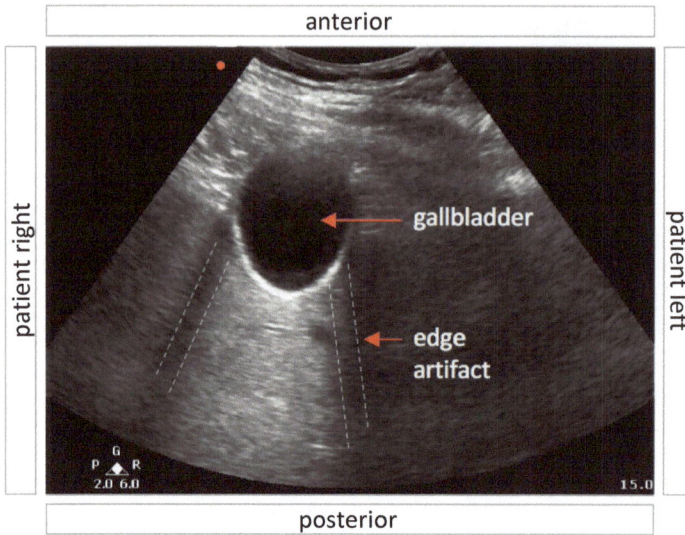

**Figure 8.9 Refraction (edge) artifact can be a false-positive for a gallstone shadow.**
The refraction artifact created by the gallbladder can be mistaken for a gallstone shadow.

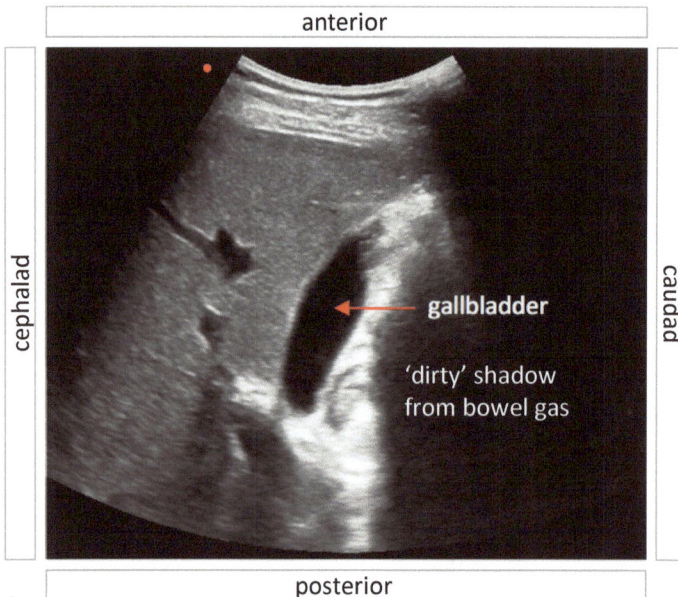

**Figure 8.10 Bowel gas can be a false-positive for a gallstone shadow.**
A 'dirty' shadow cast by bowel gas can be mistaken for a gallstone shadow. Note that shadows cast from bowel are generally diffuse and hypoechoic (grey).

**Cholecystitis sign #2. Sonographic Murphy sign**

To elicit a sonographic Murphy sign, use the subcostal approach. The probe is placed just below the ribs so that it is close to the gallbladder. As the patient breathes in, the gallbladder descends and pushes against the probe tip. A positive sonographic Murphy sign is when the patient stops breathing due to pain ('inspiratory arrest').

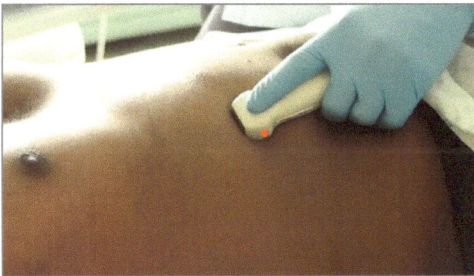

**Video 8.6 Scanning technique to elicit a positive sonographic Murphy sign with a phased array probe.**
Video: bedsideultrasoundlevel1.com

## Cholecystitis sign #3. Thickening of anterior gallbladder wall

The anterior (near-field) gallbladder wall is commonly measured in the transverse orientation. The anterior wall is less than 3 mm in thickness in a normal gallbladder.

The posterior (far-field) gallbladder wall will appear thickened due to acoustic enhancement and is thus not used for measuring wall thickness.

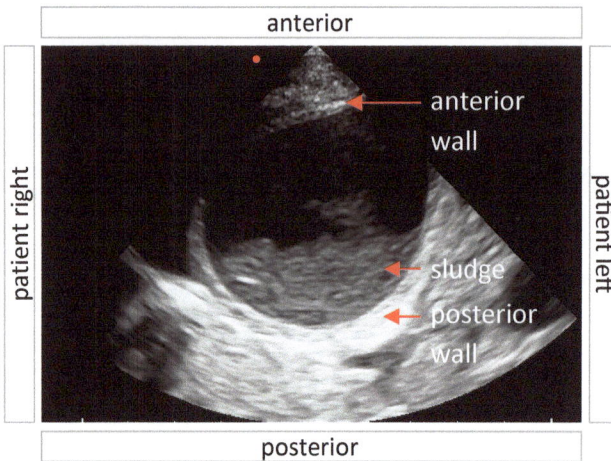

**Figure 8.11 Anterior and posterior wall of the gallbladder.**
Note that gallbladder sludge (thickened bile) does not cast a shadow.

Thickening of the anterior gallbladder wall greater than 3 mm can be seen in cholecystitis. It is also associated with other conditions [36, 37]:

- Hypoproteinemia
- Cirrhosis
- Congestive heart failure
- Hepatitis
- Renal failure
- Ascites
- Postprandial state

## Cholecystitis sign #4. Pericholecystic fluid

Fluid around the gallbladder is called pericholecystic fluid. Only a minority of cases of cholecystitis will demonstrate pericholecystic fluid, therefore it is not a sensitive sign for identifying cholecystitis. Pericholecystic fluid is quite specific for cholecystitis, but beware: it can also be seen in patients with ascites who do not have cholecystitis.

## Cholecystitis sign #5: Gallbladder distension

Normal gallbladder dimensions are 10 cm in the long orientation and 4 cm in the short orientation. Cholecystitis can result in increased gallbladder dimensions.

## Summary - Clinical relevance for cholecystitis

In a patient with right upper quadrant abdominal pain suspected of having cholecystitis:

- The presence of a positive sonographic Murphy sign has a positive predictive value of 43-72% for cholecystitis [38, 39]

- The combination of a positive sonographic Murphy sign and gallstones has a positive predictive value of 92% for cholecystitis [40]

- Gallstones combined with an anterior gallbladder wall thickness greater than 3 mm has a positive predictive value of 95% for cholecystitis [40].

## 8.4 Troubleshooting tips

- In Scanning technique #1, the gallbladder is generally found in the mid-clavicular line but can also be found anywhere between the epigastrium and the right mid-axillary line

- In cases where the gallbladder is difficult to image, having the patient breathe in and hold their breath can descend the gallbladder into the ultrasound field

- The gallbladder contracts after a patient has eaten and is thus best visualized in a fasting patient

- The shadowing caused by air in the duodenum can sometimes be mistaken for a gallstone shadow

- Examine the patient before scanning as a RUQ scar could indicate a previous cholecystectomy (surgical removal of the gallbladder)

- A short orientation view of both the gallbladder and a vessel will appear as an anechoic circle. To differentiate between the two, use color Doppler. A vessel will demonstrate flow, the gallbladder will not.

## 8.5 False-positives and false-negatives

**False-positives** (for gallstone shadows):

- **Refraction (edge) artifact:** Refraction artifacts created by the gallbladder can mimic a gallstone shadow (Figure 8.9)

- **Bowel gas:** Bowel gas casts a shadow into the far-field that can resemble a gallstone shadow. Shadows cast from bowel are generally diffuse and hypoechoic and are referred to as 'dirty' shadows. Gallstone shadows are well delineated and anechoic and referred to as 'clean' shadows.

**False-negatives** (for gallstone shadows):

- Small gallstones measuring less than 4 mm may not cast a shadow. In this situation, a shadow can sometimes be appreciated by increasing the frequency of the ultrasound.

## 8.6 CPoCUS documentation standards

The Canadian Point of Care Ultrasound Society (CPoCUS) recommends that POCUS exams be documented as follows:

- **Gallstones (GS):**
  - Negative study:       GS –
  - Positive study:       GS +
  - Indeterminate:       GS indeterminate

**Case closed:**

The 60 year old obese man with postprandial abdominal pain has gallstones and a positive sonographic Murphy sign on ultrasound examination. Cholecystitis is suspected, and he is referred to a surgeon for further care.

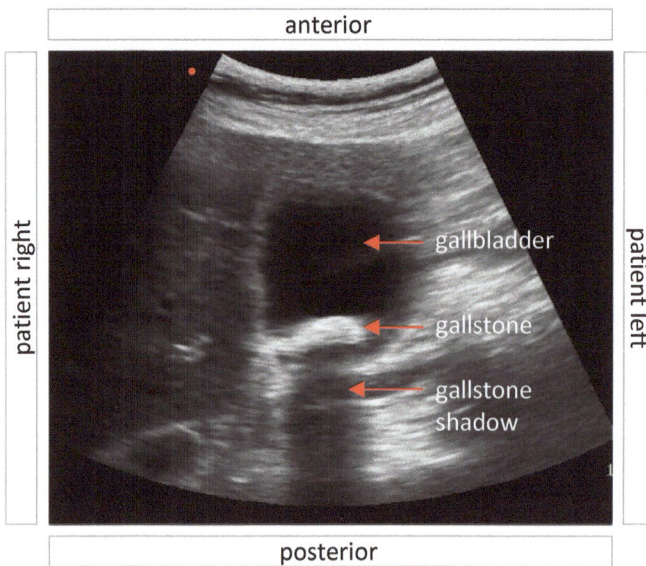

Figure 8.12 The gallbladder in transverse orientation showing a gallstone and its shadow.

# 9. KIDNEY INJURY

9.1  Probe choice

9.2  Patient position and scanning technique

9.3  Obstructive causes of kidney injury

9.4  Troubleshooting tips

9.5  CPoCUS documentation standards

**Case scenario:**

An 80 year old man presents himself to your office with generalized weakness and dyspnea. He notes decreased urine output over several weeks. On exam, the patient has pitting edema of the lower extremities and a fullness in the suprapubic area. His serum creatinine level was normal six months ago but is now high at 365 μmol/L.

**Impression:**

Acute kidney injury, rule out obstructive cause.

One cause of **kidney injury** is an obstruction to urine flow between the kidney and urethra. This type of kidney injury is called **post-renal failure**, and can be identified using bedside ultrasound [41]. This chapter will review the technique for imaging the kidney and bladder, and illustrate how to diagnose post-renal failure. Bedside ultrasound can also help to indicate whether the kidney injury is acute or chronic.

## 9.1 Probe choice

In order to image the kidney and bladder, use a low frequency phased array probe or a curvilinear probe in the abdominal setting. Low frequency probes provide the depth penetration needed to image deep structures like the kidney and bladder.

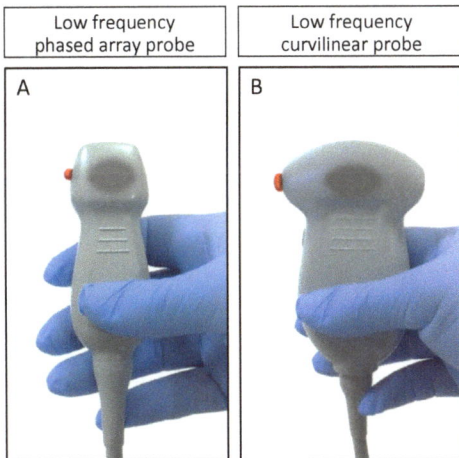

**Figure 9.1 Low frequency probes that can be used to assess a patient with kidney injury.**
**A.** A phased array probe.
**B.** A curvilinear probe.
Red circle denotes orientation marker.

## 9.2 Patient position and scanning technique

### Imaging the kidney in the coronal plane

The patient can be examined in the supine position. Because the kidney is located posteriorly, it can also be imaged with the patient in the posterior oblique position (left posterior oblique to image right kidney and vice versa). Look for the kidney with the probe in the posterior axillary line approximately level with the xiphoid. The orientation marker on the probe is pointing cephalad and slightly posteriorly.

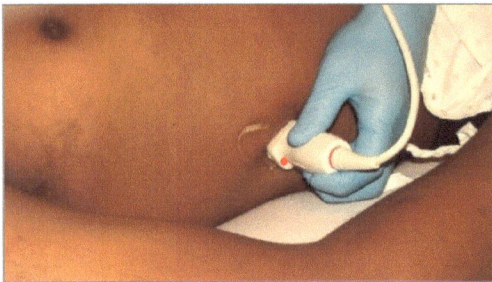

**Figure 9.2 Scanning technique for imaging the right kidney in the coronal plane with a phased array probe.**
The probe is in the coronal plane with the orientation marker pointing cephalad.

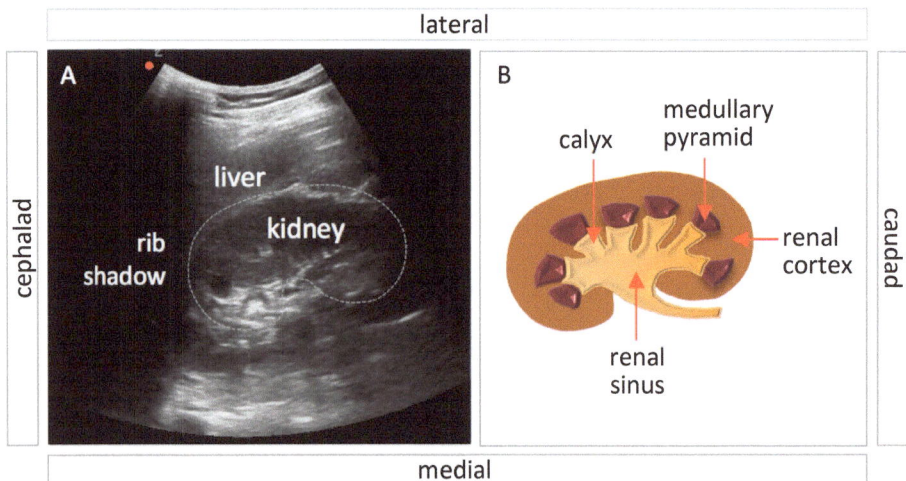

**Figure 9.3 The kidney imaged in the coronal plane.**
**A+B.** Ultrasound image (A) and corresponding schematic (B).

To image the entire kidney in the coronal plane, sweep the ultrasound beam antero-posteriorly.

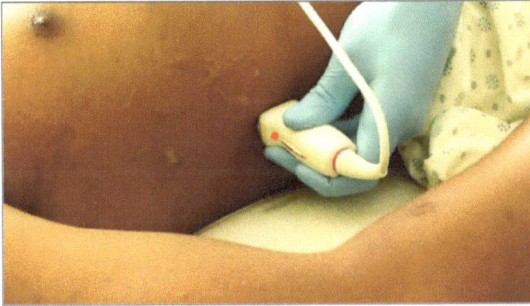

**Video 9.1 Scanning technique for imaging the entire kidney in the coronal plane.**
Video:
bedsideultrasoundlevel1.com

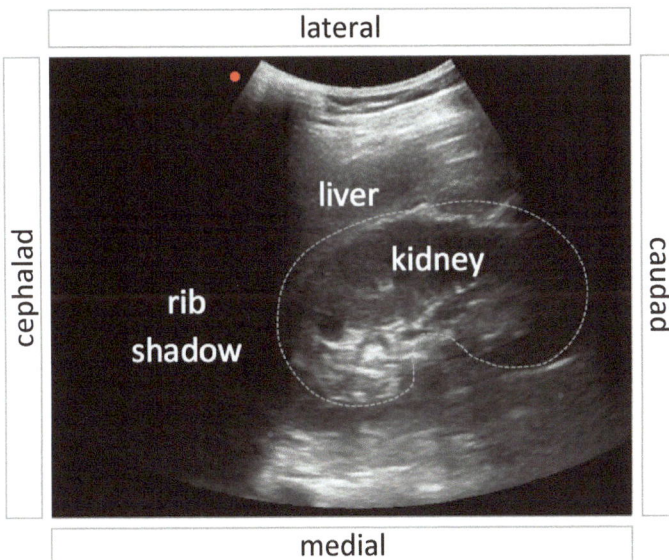

**Video 9.2 The kidney imaged in the coronal plane while sweeping the probe antero-posteriorly.**
Note that cortex of kidney is normally slightly darker than liver or spleen.
Video: bedsideultrasoundlevel1.com

Imaging the kidney in the transverse plane

Once the kidney has been located in the coronal plane, turn the probe so that the orientation marker points to the patient's right. This adjustment provides an image of the kidney in the transverse plane. To image the entire kidney in the transverse plane, sweep the ultrasound beam from upper to lower pole.

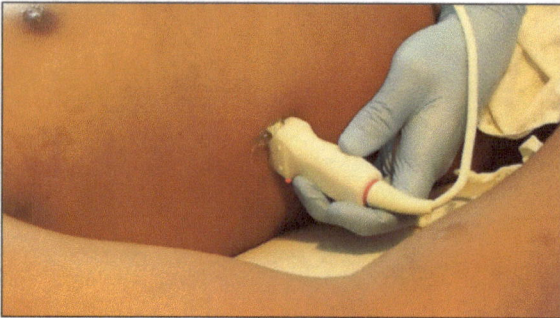

**Video 9.3 Scanning technique for imaging the right kidney in the transverse plane from upper to lower pole.**
Sweep the probe from cephalad to caudad. Video: bedsideultrasoundlevel1.com

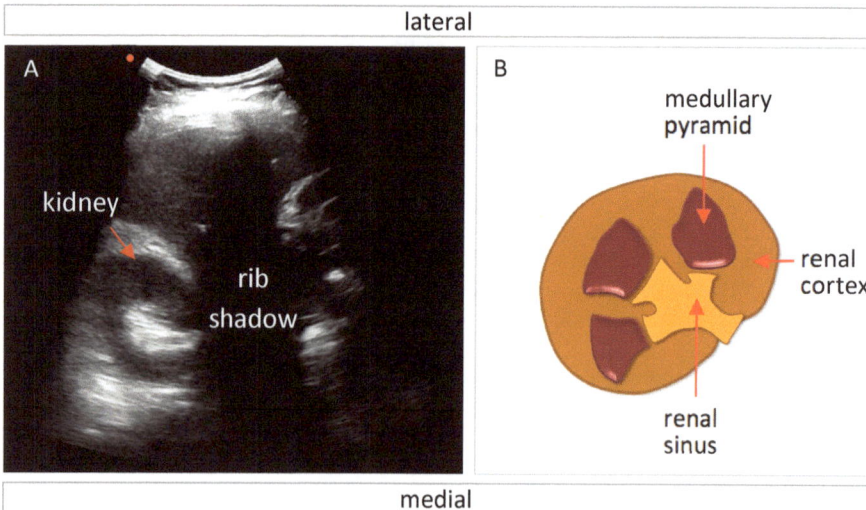

**Video 9.4 The kidney imaged in the transverse plane while sweeping the probe from cephalad to caudad.**
**A+B.** Ultrasound image (A) and corresponding schematic (B).
Video: bedsideultrasoundlevel1.com

## Imaging the bladder in the sagittal plane

To image the bladder in the sagittal plane, place the probe just above the symphysis pubis, with the orientation marker pointing cephalad. Rock the probe in order to point the probe caudally. The urine in the bladder appears anechoic (black).

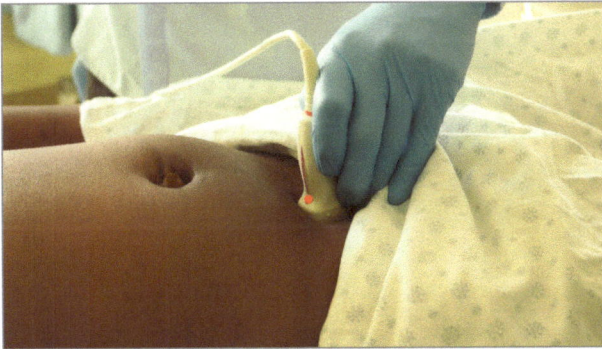

**Figure 9.4 Scanning technique for imaging the bladder in the sagittal plane.**

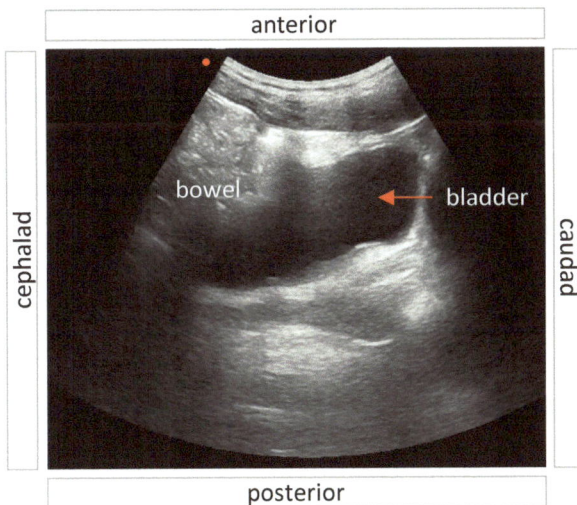

**Figure 9.5 The male bladder imaged in the sagittal plane.**

## Imaging the bladder in the transverse plane

To image the bladder in the transverse plane, place the probe just above the symphysis pubis, with the orientation marker pointing to the patient's right. Point the probe caudally.

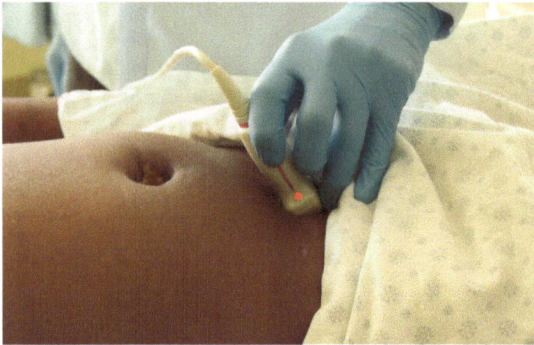

Figure 9.6 Scanning technique for imaging the bladder in the transverse plane.

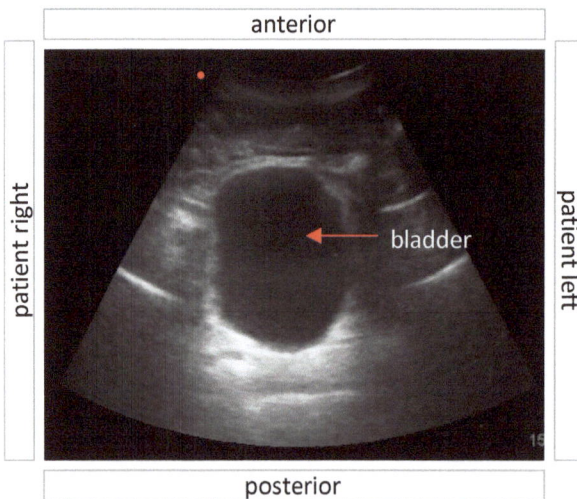

Figure 9.7 The male bladder in the transverse plane.

## 9.3  Obstructive causes of kidney injury

Ultrasound is useful in identifying obstructive causes of kidney injury (post-renal failure). Hydronephrosis and a distended post-void bladder are ultrasonographic signs of obstruction to urinary flow.

### Clinical relevance - Hydronephrosis

Hydronephrosis is a distension of the renal sinus and calyces due to an obstruction of the urinary tract distal to the kidney [42].

Unilateral hydronephrosis is generally due to pathology of the ureter or ureterovesicular junction (e.g. urolithiasis).

Bilateral hydronephrosis is generally due to pathology at the level of the bladder (e.g. bladder tumor, neurogenic bladder) or distal to the bladder (e.g. prostatic disease).

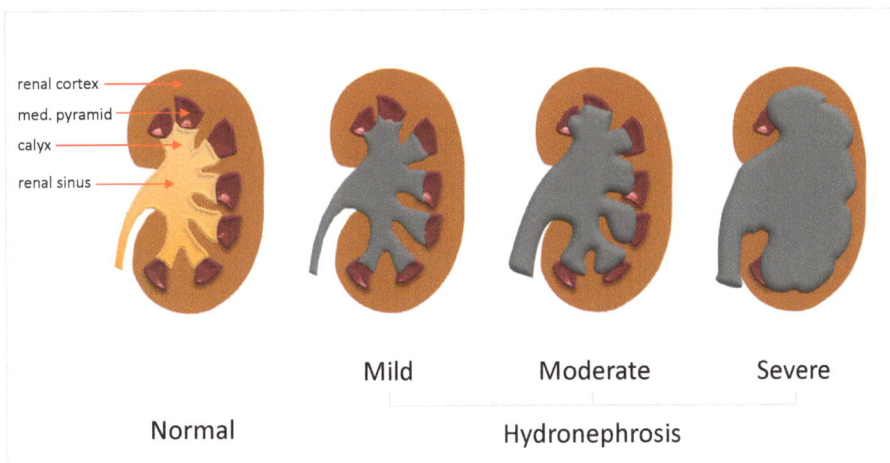

**Figure 9.8 Schematic depicting grades of hydronephrosis.**

Mild:             Distension of collecting system (renal sinus and calyces).
Moderate:     Increased distension of the collecting system.
Severe:         Ballooning of calyces with cortical thinning.

In hydronephrosis, the calyces and renal sinus appear anechoic (black) and distended on the ultrasound image.

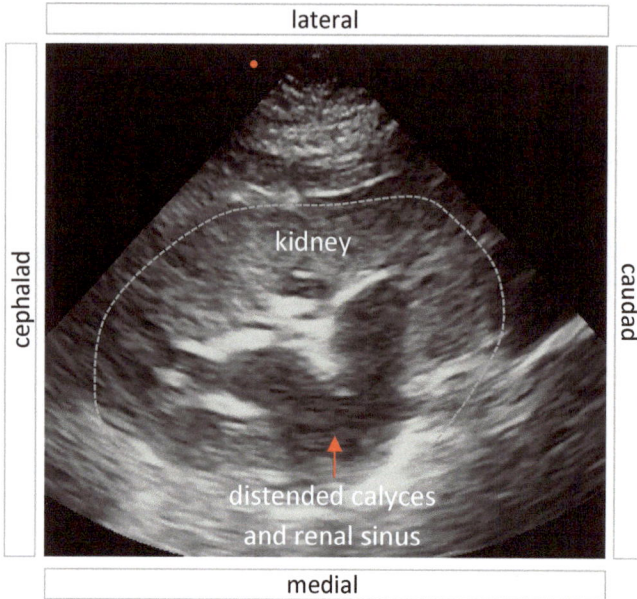

**Figure 9.9 The kidney in the coronal plane with moderate hydronephrosis, i.e. 'the bear paw sign'.**

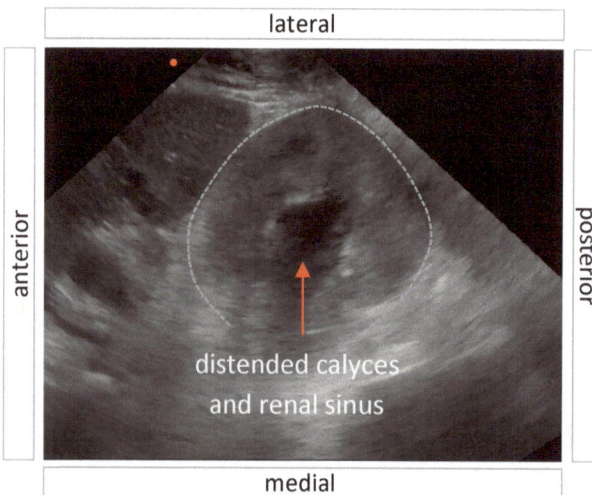

**Figure 9.10 The left kidney in the transverse plane with moderate hydronephrosis.**

**Clinical relevance - Post-void bladder volume**

The upper limit of normal **post-void bladder volume** is 50-100 ml in an adult patient [43]. However, in patients with chronic incomplete emptying of the bladder, this value can be much higher without associated kidney injury.

Although many portable ultrasound machines have a pre-programmed formula for calculating bladder volume, a gross estimate of post-void bladder volume can be determined using the following formula [44].

---

**Bladder volume (ml) = 0.75 x ($W_{trans}$ x $H_{trans}$ x $L_{sagit}$)**

$W_{trans}$  = maximum width in transverse plane (cm)

$H_{trans}$  = maximum height in transverse plane (cm)

$L_{sagit}$  = maximum length in sagittal plane (cm)

---

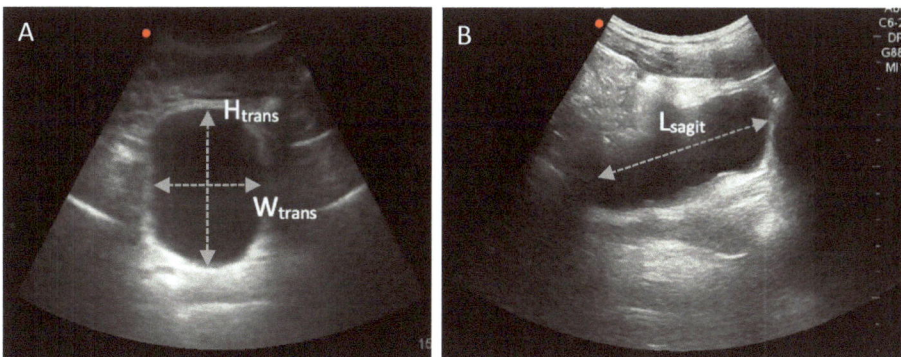

**Figure 9.11 Gross estimation of bladder volume.**
**A.** Maximum bladder height (Htrans) and width (Wtrans) in transverse plane.
**B.** Maximum bladder length (Lsagit) in sagittal plane.

The assessment of post-void bladder volume is clinically relevant in the following common scenarios:

- A patient presents with kidney injury and is found to have a high post-void residual bladder volume. In an older male patient, this condition is commonly due to prostatic disease

- A patient with a **Foley catheter** stops urinating. If there is a full bladder on ultrasound, then the diagnosis is a blocked or misplaced Foley catheter.

**Table 9.1 Combined kidney and bladder ultrasound findings, and common associated pathologies**

| | | Ultrasound findings | |
|---|---|---|---|
| | | **Post-void bladder volume** | |
| | | **Increased volume** | **Normal volume** |
| **Ultrasound findings** **Kidney - Hydronephrosis** | | Pathology at the level of the bladder: <br><br> • neurogenic bladder <br> • medications <br><br><br> Pathology distal to the bladder: <br><br> • prostatic disease <br> • blocked Foley | Pathology between kidney and ureterovesicular junction: <br><br> • bladder tumor <br> • urolithiasis <br> • ureteral tumor |

## Clinical relevance - Acute vs. chronic kidney injury

The cortex of the kidney is normally of darker echogenicity than the solid organ located cephalad to the kidney. Note that the liver is the solid organ cephalad to the right kidney while the spleen is the solid organ cephalad to the left kidney. In acute kidney injury, this echogenicity relationship remains unchanged. In chronic kidney injury, the kidney cortex often takes on a brighter echogenicity. In extreme cases, the cortex can be brighter than the solid organ located cephalad. Therefore, if a patient presents suffering kidney injury and the kidney cortex is darker than the organ cephalad, the kidney injury is likely acute. If a patient presents suffering kidney injury and the kidney cortex is the same echogenicity or a brighter echogenicity than the organ located cephalad, the kidney injury is likely chronic. In chronic kidney injury, the kidney is also generally smaller (normal kidney length is between 9-13 cm).

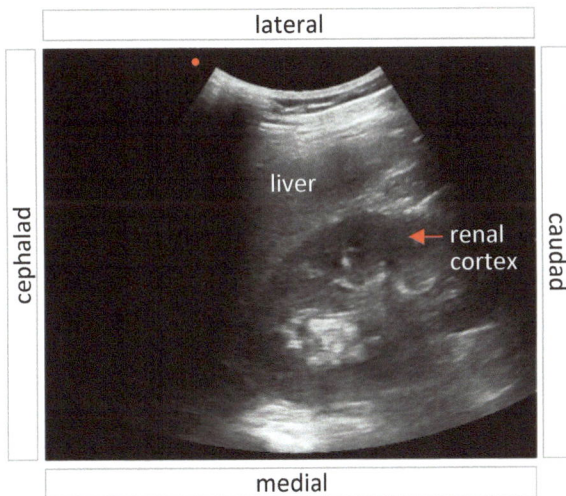

**Figure 9.12 Acute kidney injury.**
Note that the echotexture of the right kidney cortex is darker than the liver located cephalad, as for normal patients, thus suggesting acute kidney injury.

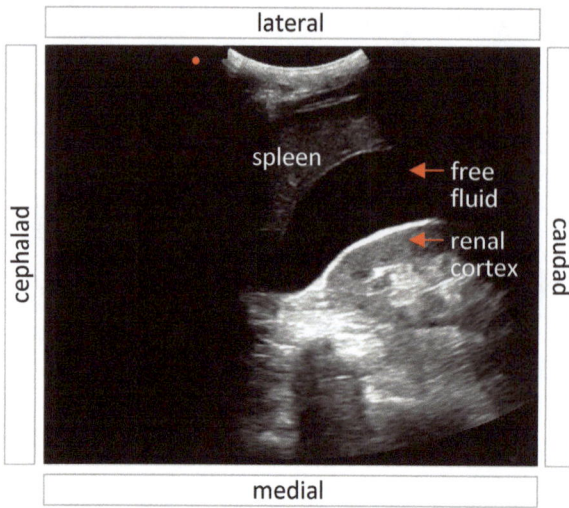

**Figure 9.13 Chronic kidney injury.**
Note that the cortex of the left kidney is a brighter echogenicity than the spleen located cephalad (partly due in this case to the enhancement artifact caused by free fluid).

## Clinical relevance - Other pathology

Kidney cysts are a common finding. To differentiate a kidney cyst from hydronephrosis, note that the cyst is not in communication with a distended renal sinus.

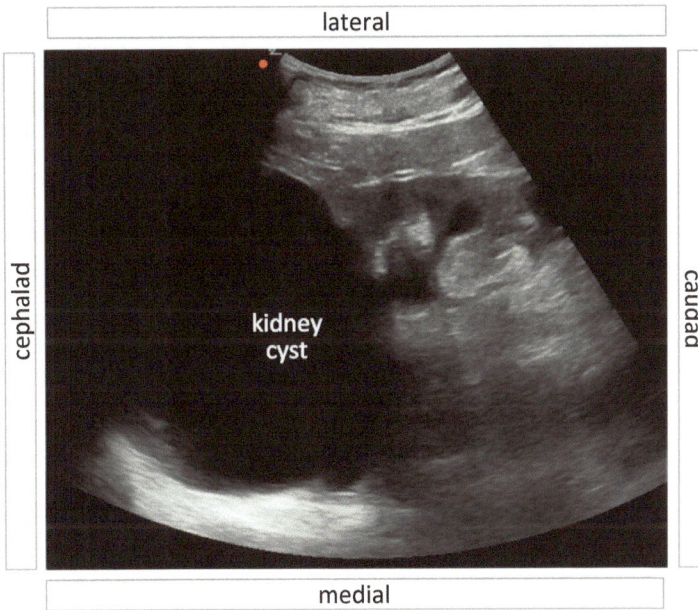

**Figure 9.14 Kidney cyst.**
Note the large upper pole kidney cyst is not in communication with the renal sinus.

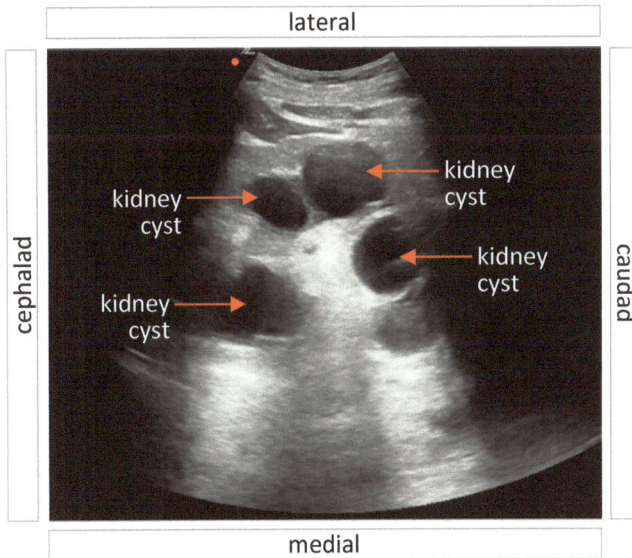

**Figure 9.15 Multiple kidney cysts.**
Note multiple kidney cysts, none of which communicate with the renal sinus.

## 9.4 Troubleshooting tips

- When rib shadows obscure the view of the kidney, ask the patient to breathe in and hold their breath. This action will cause the kidney to descend below the ribs, improving the quality of the image (*see Video 9.5*)

- To avoid rib shadows entirely, turn the probe obliquely (upper part of probe angled posteriorly) so the ultrasound beam runs along the intercostal space.

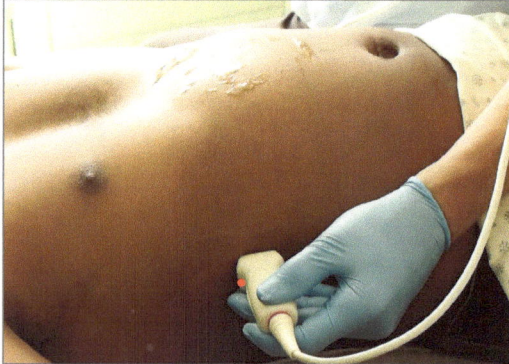

**Video 9.5 Scanning technique for removing rib shadows.**
Video:
bedsideultrasoundlevel1.com

## 9.5 CPoCUS documentation standards

The Canadian Point of Care Ultrasound Society (CPoCUS) recommends that POCUS exams be documented as follows:

- **Hydronephrosis (hydro):**
  - Negative study:      no hydro
  - Positive study:      mild-moderate hydro
                         severe hydro
  - Indeterminate:       hydro indeterminate

**Case closed:**

The 80 year old man with acute kidney injury has bilateral hydronephrosis and a full post-void bladder on ultrasound examination. Bladder outlet obstruction is suspected, a Foley catheter is placed, and a urologist is consulted.

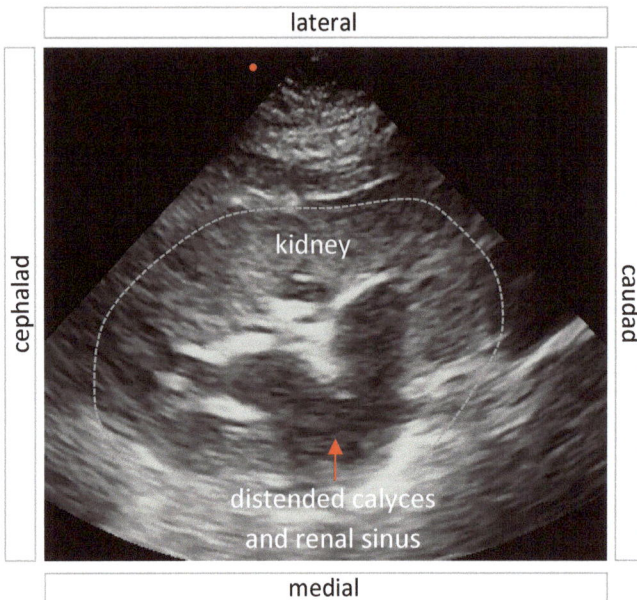

Figure 9.16 The kidney in the coronal plane with moderate hydronephrosis.

# 10. DEEP VENOUS THROMBOSIS (DVT) OF THE LOWER LIMB

10.1  Probe choice

10.2  Patient position and scanning technique - Common femoral vein

10.3  Patient position and scanning technique - Popliteal vein

10.4  Troubleshooting tips

10.5  False-positives and false-negatives

10.6  CPoCUS documentation standards

---

**Case scenario:**

A 40 year old woman with no significant past medical history presents herself to the emergency room with a swollen leg. Her only current medication is the birth control pill. She has just completed a 14 hour flight. Physical exam reveals a swollen, non-tender left leg, no cord, and negative Homan's sign.

**Impression:**

Swollen leg, high suspicion for deep venous thrombosis (DVT).

---

Traditionally, a complete lower limb venous ultrasound examination with color Doppler and compression is used for the detection of deep venous thrombosis (DVT). In this chapter, we introduce an abbreviated lower limb ultrasound examination using **compression ultrasound** only. The abbreviated examination includes imaging the common femoral vein and the popliteal vein. There is evidence to suggest that an abbreviated compression ultrasound examination of the leg is sufficiently sensitive to detect the majority of clinically significant DVTs of the lower limb in ambulatory patients [45-49].

## 10.1  Probe choice

A high frequency linear probe is used when examining veins. High frequency probes give excellent resolution of superficial structures.

In obese patients or patients with muscular legs, the vascular structures may be too deep to visualize with a high frequency probe. In these cases, a low frequency curvilinear probe can be used.

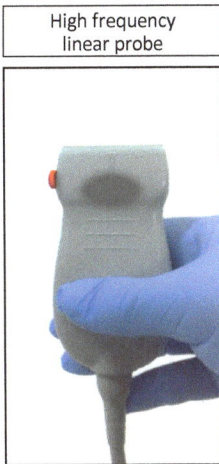

High frequency
linear probe

**Figure 10.1 A high frequency linear probe is used to assess veins of the lower leg.**
Red circle denotes orientation marker.

## 10.2 Patient position and scanning technique - Common femoral vein

Patients can be evaluated in the supine position with the head of the bed elevated to 30°, thus ensuring engorgement of the lower extremity veins. The leg should be externally rotated with the knee slightly bent.

The probe is placed just below the inguinal ligament with the orientation marker pointing towards the patient's right. This probe position will provide a transverse view of the common femoral vein. Veins appear anechoic (black) on the ultrasound image.

Scan the common femoral vein from the inguinal ligament caudally until the junction between the common femoral vein, femoral vein, and deep femoral vein.

### Clinical relevance - DVT in the common femoral vein

During compression ultrasound, the examiner compresses the vein with the ultrasound probe. If the opposing walls of the vein touch each other, a venous thrombosis is excluded at that discrete point. If a DVT is present, the opposing walls of the vein will not touch each other when the vein is compressed. A DVT can also be detected as a slightly hyperechoic (white) structure within the vein lumen [50].

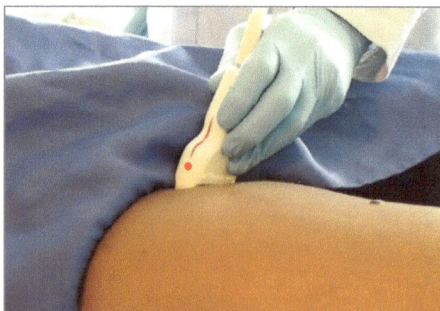

**Video 10.1 Scanning technique for compression ultrasound of the common femoral vein.**
Video: bedsideultrasoundlevel1.com

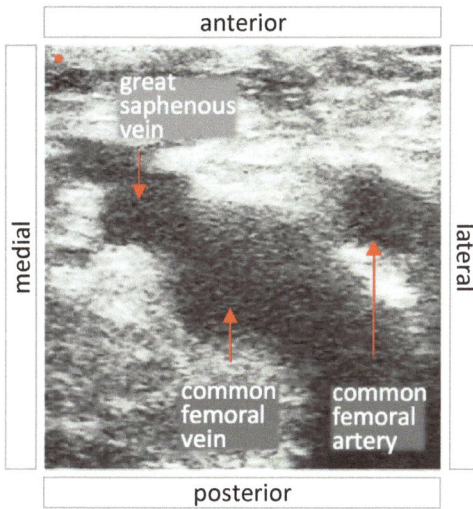

**Video 10.2 Compression ultrasound of a normal left common femoral vein.**
When the vein is compressed, the opposite walls of the vein touch each other, therefore
excluding a DVT at this point. Video: bedsideultrasoundlevel1.com

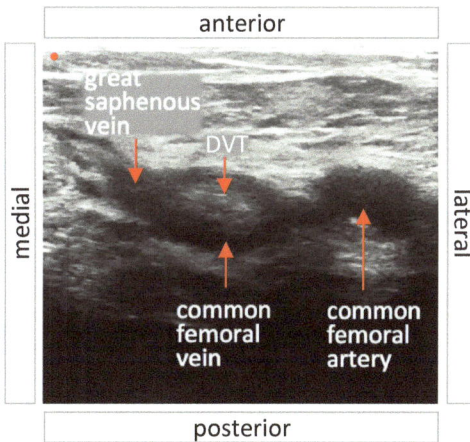

**Video 10.3 Compression ultrasound demonstrating a DVT in the left common
femoral vein.**
When the vein is compressed, the walls of the vein remain separated due to the
presence of the DVT. The DVT is hyperechoic (white) and is seen within the lumen of
the vein. Video: bedsideultrasoundlevel1.com

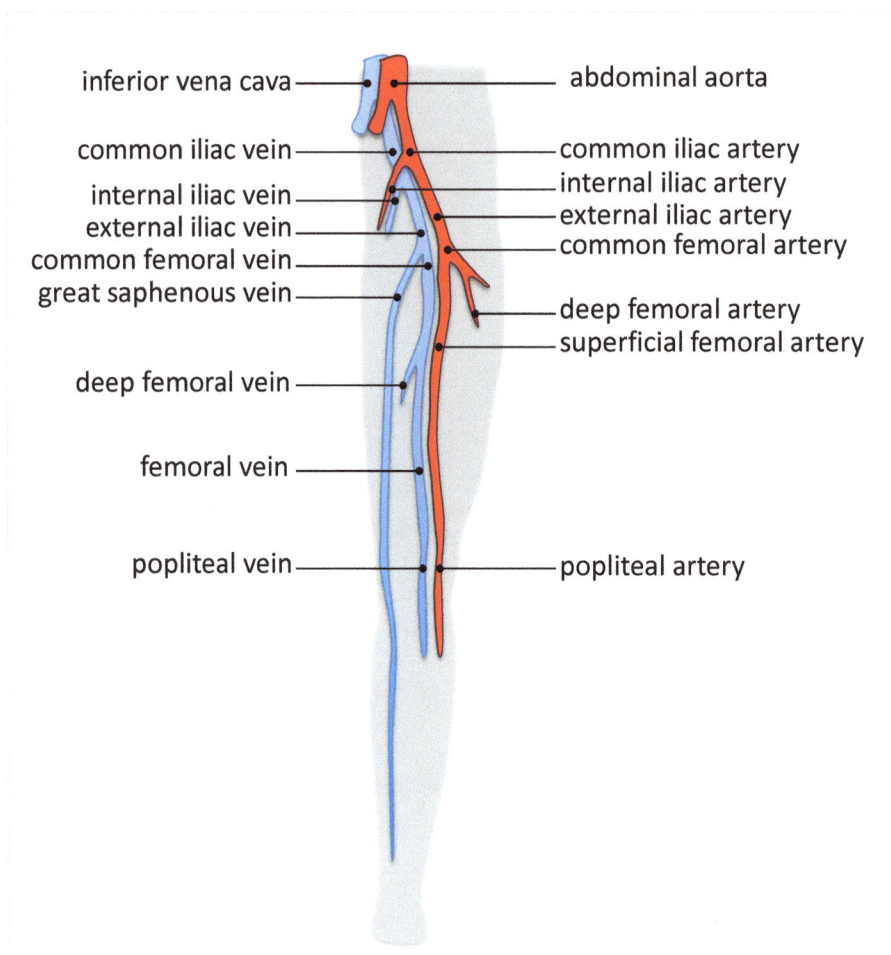

**Figure 10.2 Schematic of veins and arteries of the upper leg.**

There are usually four anatomical patterns observed when ultrasound is performed in the transverse plane between the inguinal ligament and the junction between the common femoral, femoral, and deep femoral veins.

**Table 10.1 Anatomical patterns observed from transverse ultrasound examination of the common femoral vein in the caudal direction**

| Patterns observed from examination of the common femoral vein | | |
|---|---|---|
| Pattern #1 | Junction of the great saphenous vein (GSV) with the common femoral vein (CFV). The common femoral artery (CFA) is lateral to the CFV | medial                    lateral<br>GSV<br>CFV        CFA |
| Pattern #2 | Common femoral vein (CFV) medial to bifurcation of the common femoral artery into the superficial (SFA) and deep femoral arteries (DFA) | SFA<br>CFV<br>DFA |
| Pattern #3 | The femoral vein (FV) and deep femoral vein (DFV) medial to the superficial femoral artery (SFA) | SFA<br>FV<br>DFV |
| Pattern #4 | The femoral vein (FV) posterior to the superficial femoral artery (SFA) | SFA<br>FV |

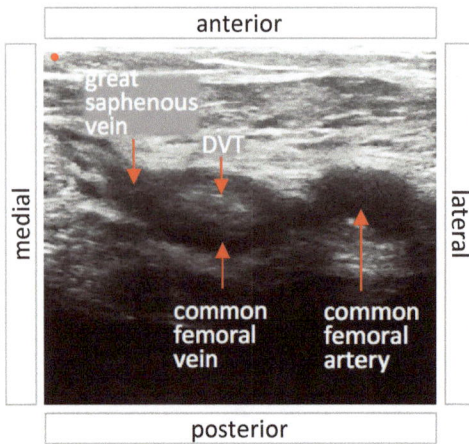

**Figure 10.3 Pattern #1: Junction of the great saphenous vein with the left common femoral vein.**
This pattern is seen immediately caudal to the inguinal ligament. The great saphenous vein enters the common femoral vein medially. The common femoral artery is lateral to the common femoral vein.

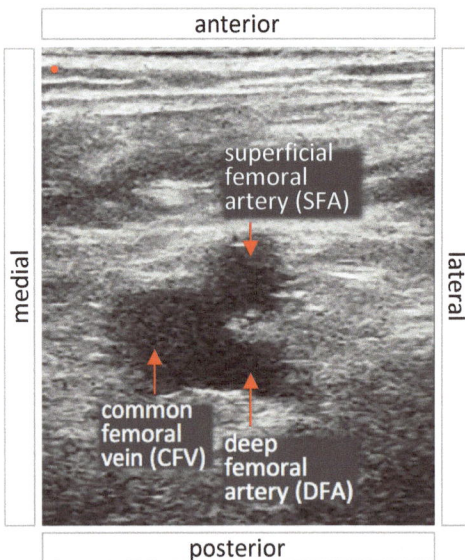

**Figure 10.4 Pattern #2: Common femoral vein medial to bifurcation of femoral artery.**
The common femoral artery bifurcates several centimeters caudal to Pattern #1.

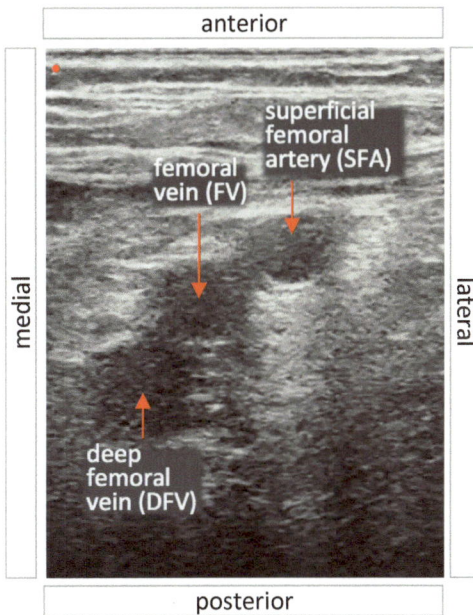

**Figure 10.5 Pattern #3: The femoral vein and deep femoral vein medial to the superficial femoral artery.**
The deep femoral artery is no longer visible.

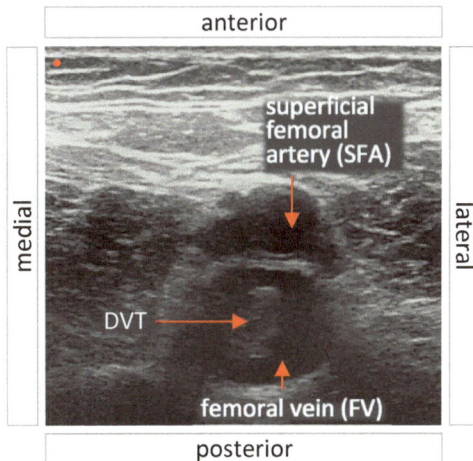

**Figure 10.6 Pattern #4: The femoral vein posterior to the superficial femoral artery.**
The deep femoral vein is no longer visible. The hyperechoic (white) structure within the femoral vein is a DVT.

Once compression ultrasound has been completed 2 cm distal to the junction between the femoral and deep femoral veins, leave the upper leg and proceed to examine the popliteal vein on the same leg (see next section).

## 10.3   Patient position and scanning technique - Popliteal vein

The popliteal vein can be examined with the patient in several different positions. If the patient is not mobile, examine the popliteal vein with the patient lying in the supine position, the hips externally rotated, and knees slightly bent. The head of the bed is elevated to 30° to ensure the leg veins are engorged with blood. Alternatively, the patient can lie on their side with knees bent. If the patient is mobile, the patient can be examined prone with the knee slightly bent by placing a pillow under the dorsum of the foot. Mobile patients can also be examined while sitting on the edge of the bed. Due to the different patient positions, the convention is to point the probe orientation marker to the lateral side of the patient which provides a transverse image of the popliteal vein.

Compression ultrasound of the popliteal vein is performed at every centimeter from the proximal popliteal fossa until the calf. To find the proximal point of the fossa to begin the scan, first find the popliteal vein in the popliteal fossa. The popliteal vein will be near-field to the popliteal artery. Then slide your probe proximally and note that the popliteal vein moves progressively into the far-field. This is where the popliteal scan starts.

At the calf, the popliteal vein divides into the anterior tibial and the tibioperoneal trunk (the popliteal vein trifurcates). At this point, the examiner will note multiple smaller vessels originating from the popliteal vein. The examination of the popliteal vein is complete two centimeters distal to its trifurcation.

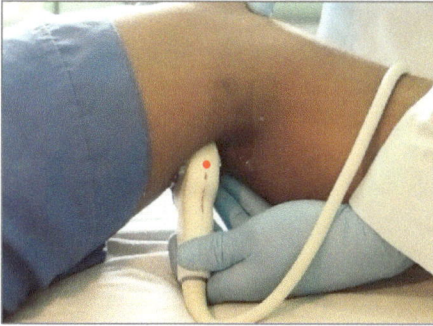

**Video 10.4 Scanning technique for compression ultrasound of the popliteal vein with patient supine.**
Video: bedsideultrasoundlevel1.com

## Clinical relevance - DVT in the popliteal vein

During compression ultrasound of the popliteal vein, the examiner compresses the vein with the ultrasound probe. If the opposing walls of the vein touch each other, a venous thrombosis is excluded at that discrete point. If a DVT is present, the opposing walls of the vein will not touch each other when the vein is compressed.

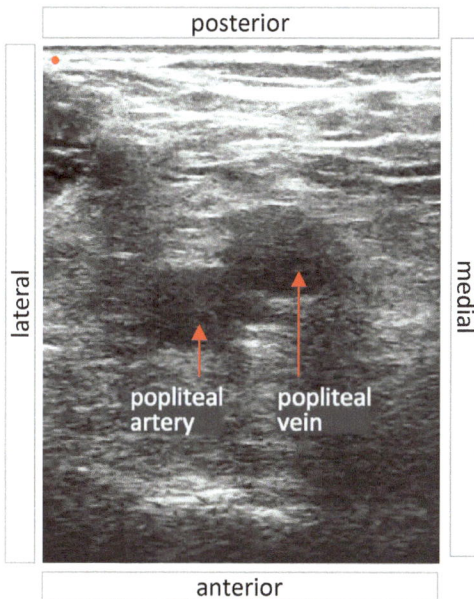

**Video 10.5 Compression ultrasound of a normal popliteal vein.**
The popliteal vein collapses when compressed, excluding a DVT at this point. The artery does not collapse when compressed. Video: bedsideultrasoundlevel1.com

## 10.4   Troubleshooting tips

- To better visualize the popliteal vein, the patient may be examined while sitting or in a prone position

- Anatomic variance: There may be two popliteal veins in the same leg

- In obese patients with swollen legs, lowering the frequency of the probe increases depth penetration and may improve the quality of the image

- The femoral vein is sometimes referred to as the superficial femoral vein. This can be confusing as a thrombus in this vein is considered a DVT.

## 10.5 False-positives and false-negatives

**False-positives (for a DVT):**

- **Lymph nodes:** Lymph nodes appear hyperechoic and non-compressible as does a DVT. However, as the probe is rotated ninety degrees, it will be clear that the structure (node) is a sphere and not the tubular structure seen with a vessel

- **Superficial thrombophlebitis:** Superficial thrombophlebitis appears as a thrombosis within a superficial vein. This inflammatory process can present with leg swelling and tenderness but have different management than DVT

- **Baker's cyst:** A Baker's cyst can present with leg swelling and pain behind the knee, and appears in the popliteal fossa as an anechoic non-compressible structure which can be mistaken for DVT. However, it will have no flow apparent on Doppler

- **Chronic DVT:** A chronic DVT will appear hyperechoic and non-compressible. Sometimes there will be flow (recanalization) through the center of the thrombus. Ask for a history of DVT in that leg.

**False-negatives (for a DVT):**

- **Inadequate scanning area:** Be sure that the entire area described above has been scanned. Thrombi can be small and missed by an inadequate scan

- **Inadequate images due to leg edema or obesity**: To improve image quality in this situation, try lowering the frequency on the probe or consider using a low frequency curvilinear probe in extreme cases

- **Duplicate popliteal veins:** A significant percentage of people have two popliteal veins. Be sure to scan both! One may be normal and the other may have a DVT

- **DVT in the pelvis:** A DVT in the pelvis will not be seen on the scans described in this chapter. If your clinical suspicion suggests DVT always ask for a formal scan by an imaging specialist.

## 10.6 CPoCUS documentation standards

The Canadian Point of Care Ultrasound Society (CPoCUS) recommends that POCUS exams be documented as follows:

- **Deep venous thrombosis (DVT):**

  o Negative study:     DVT −

  o Positive study:      DVT +

  o Indeterminate:      DVT indeterminate

**Case closed:**

The 40 year old woman with a swollen leg has a hyperechoic (grey) structure within the common femoral vein on ultrasound examination. The vein does not collapse completely on compression ultrasound, suggesting a DVT. Appropriate anti-coagulation is ordered.

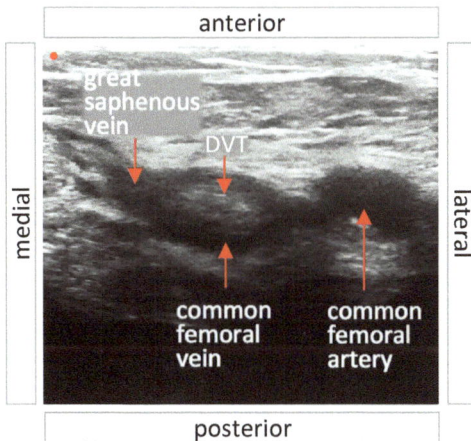

Figure 10.7 A DVT within the lumen of the left common femoral vein.

# 11. ECTOPIC PREGNANCY

11.1  Probe choice

11.2  Patient position and scanning technique

11.3  Criteria for diagnosing an intra-uterine pregnancy

11.4  Troubleshooting tips

11.5  False-positives and false-negatives

11.6  CPoCUS documentation standards

**Case scenario:**

A 30 year old woman with a history of pelvic inflammatory disease presents herself to your rural clinic with vaginal bleeding and pelvic pain. Her LMP was seven or eight weeks ago. Her vital signs are stable. A qualitative urinary BHCG test is positive.

**Impression:**

Rule out ectopic pregnancy.

The goal of this chapter is to introduce the use of trans-abdominal pelvic ultrasound as an adjunct in the assessment of a patient with a possible ectopic pregnancy.

An ectopic pregnancy is the presence of an extra-uterine pregnancy. Ectopic pregnancies are potentially life-threatening due to their tendency to rupture and cause bleeding. A clinician must consider ectopic pregnancy in a pregnant woman with abdominal pain or vaginal bleeding during the first trimester. Ectopic pregnancy can be excluded by demonstrating that the pregnancy is intra-uterine on point-of-care ultrasound.

## 11.1   Probe choice

In order to image the female pelvis use a phased array probe in the abdominal setting or a low frequency curvilinear probe. Low frequency probes provide the depth penetration needed to image deep structures like the uterus.

Transvaginal ultrasound technique and probes will not be discussed in this introductory book.

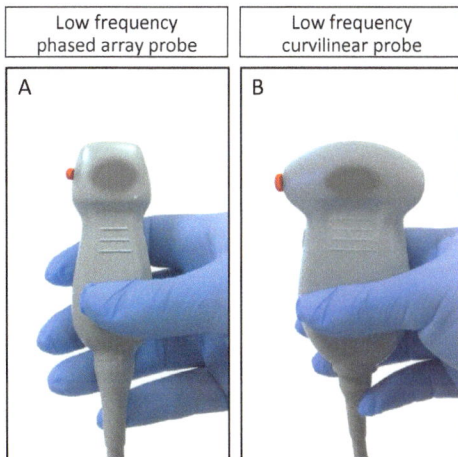

**Figure 11.1 Low frequency probes that can be used to assess a patient with suspected ectopic pregnancy.**
**A.** A phased array probe.
**B.** A curvilinear probe.
Red circle denotes orientation marker.

## 11.2   Patient position and scanning technique

The patient is examined in the supine position with a full bladder. Start by scanning the patient in the sagittal plane, followed by the transverse plane.

### Imaging the uterus in the sagittal plane

To scan the uterus in the sagittal plane, place the probe just above the symphysis pubis with the orientation marker pointing cephalad. Rock the probe caudally. To ensure complete imaging of the uterus, sweep the probe by 45° to the right and left while in the sagittal plane.

The uterus appears as a hypoechoic (grey) pear-shaped structure below the bladder. An important landmark in the non-pregnant uterus is the **endometrial stripe**. The endometrial stripe appears as a hyperechoic (white) line in the center of the uterus.

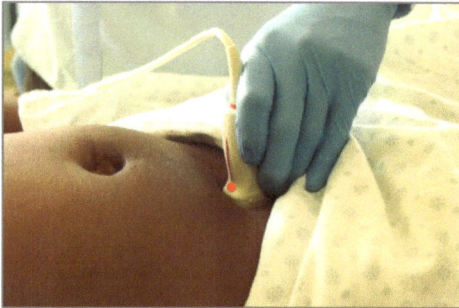

**Figure 11.2 Scanning technique for imaging the uterus in the sagittal plane using a phased array probe.**

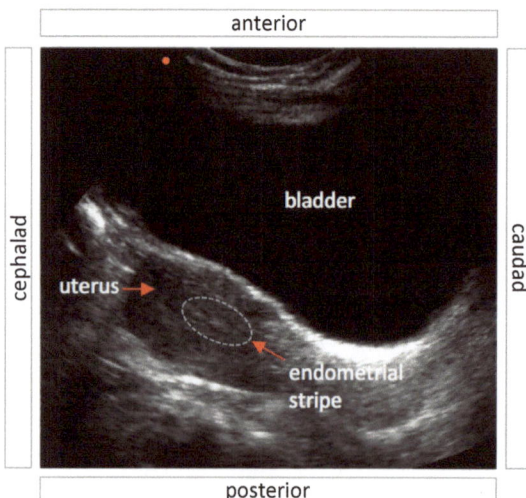

**Figure 11.3 The female pelvis imaged in the sagittal plane.**

## Imaging the uterus in the transverse plane

The uterus is a mobile organ and thus rarely lies exactly at the midline. To scan the uterus in the transverse plane, place the probe just above the symphysis pubis with the orientation marker pointing to the patient's right. Sweep the probe caudally. To ensure complete imaging of the uterus, scan from the fundus to the cervix in the transverse plane.

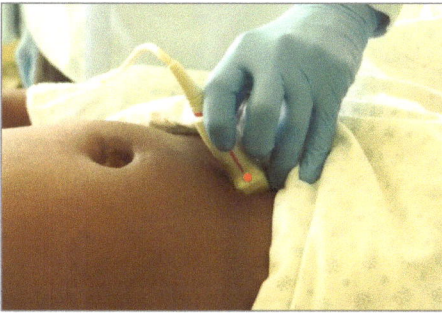

**Figure 11.4 Scanning technique for imaging the uterus in the transverse plane using a phased array probe.**

The uterus appears as a hypoechoic (grey) round structure below the bladder. The **endometrial stripe** is visible at the center of the uterus.

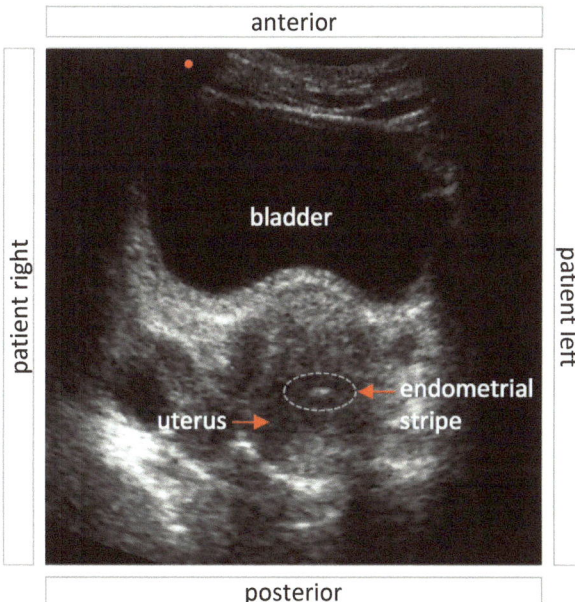

**Figure 11.5 The female pelvis imaged in the transverse plane.**

## 11.3  Criteria for diagnosing an intra-uterine pregnancy (IUP)

There are five ultrasound criteria necessary for diagnosis of an intra-uterine pregnancy (IUP) [30, 51-54].

Three criteria are necessary to diagnose pregnancy and they must all be imaged within the uterus:

- Criteria #1:  Gestational sac
- Criteria #2:  Yolk sac or fetal pole within the gestational sac
- Criteria #3:  Decidual reaction around the gestational sac.

Two criteria are necessary to confirm the identity of the uterus and establish that the pregnancy is intra-uterine:

- Criteria #4:  Bladder uterine juxtaposition
- Criteria #5:  Myometrial mantle of at least 5mm.

**Criteria #1: Gestational sac.** The first sign of an intra-uterine pregnancy on the ultrasound image is a gestational sac. The gestational sac appears at 5-6 weeks gestational age on trans-abdominal pelvic ultrasound as an anechoic (black) area within the uterus. The presence of a gestational sac alone is insufficient for diagnosing an intra-uterine pregnancy because a 'pseudogestational sac' within the uterus appears in approximately 5% of ectopic pregnancies.

**Criteria #2:** A **yolk sac** appears as an anechoic (black) structure surrounded by a hyperechoic (white) membrane between 6-7 weeks gestation on trans-abdominal pelvic ultrasound. The yolk sac is a thin-walled round structure located within the gestational sac. A **fetal pole** appears between 7-8 weeks gestation on trans-abdominal pelvic ultrasound. The fetal pole appears as a hyperechoic (white) structure next to the yolk sac.

**Criteria #3: Decidual reaction** is a hyperechoic (white) region surrounding the gestational sac.

Because an ectopic pregnancy may have a visible <u>extra-uterine</u> gestational and yolk sac, we also require two criteria to be sure the pregnancy is intra-uterine.

**Criteria #4: Bladder uterine juxtaposition** means that the bladder and the uterus are immediately next to each other on the ultrasound image. The juxtaposition ensures that the uterus is properly identified. The pregnancy must be clearly imaged within the uterus.

**Criteria #5: Myometrial mantle** of at least 5 mm in all areas between the gestational sac and the outer wall of the uterus. An ectopic pregnancy at the junction between the uterus and fallopian tube (interstitial or cornual pregnancy) will have a thin wall of myometrium between the gestational sac and the outer wall of the uterus. At least 5 mm of myometrial mantle ensures that the pregnancy is intra-uterine.

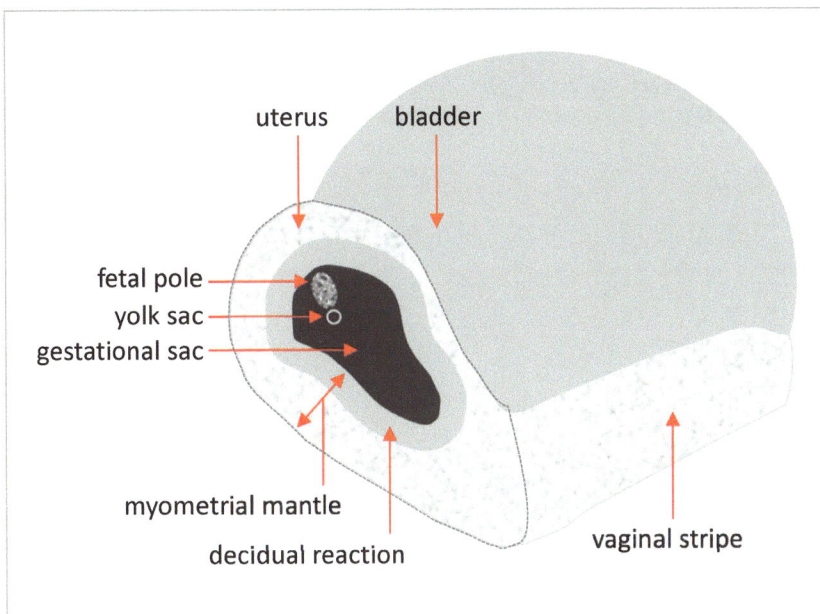

**Figure 11.6 Schematic showing criteria for intra-uterine pregnancy in the trans-abdominal sagittal view.**
Note that the bladder and the uterus are directly juxtaposed.

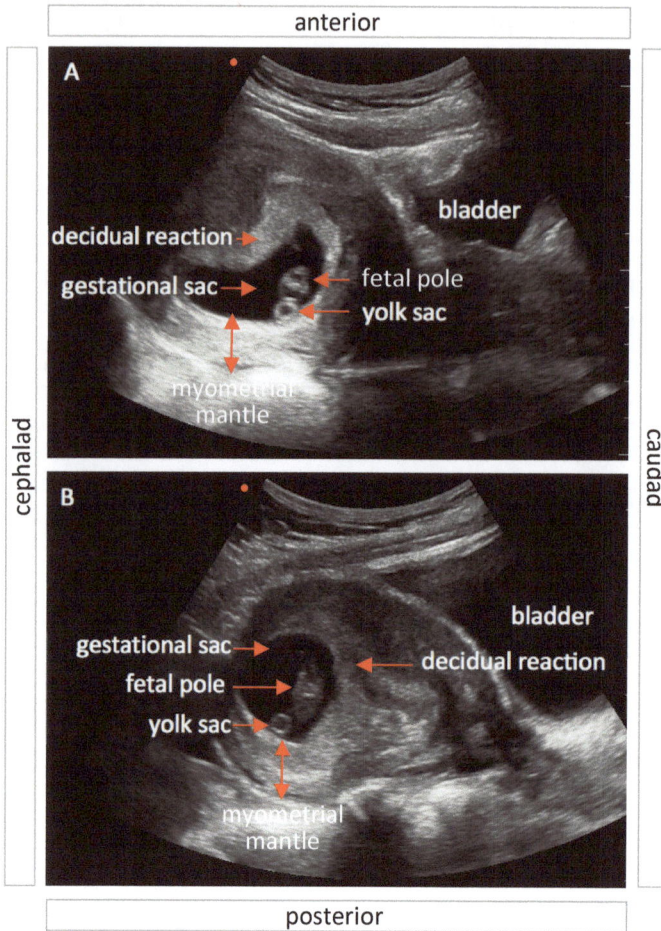

**Figure 11.7 Gestational sac, yolk sac, and fetal pole imaged within the uterus in the sagittal plane.**
**A+B.** Two examples of female pelvis showing criteria for intra-uterine pregnancy.

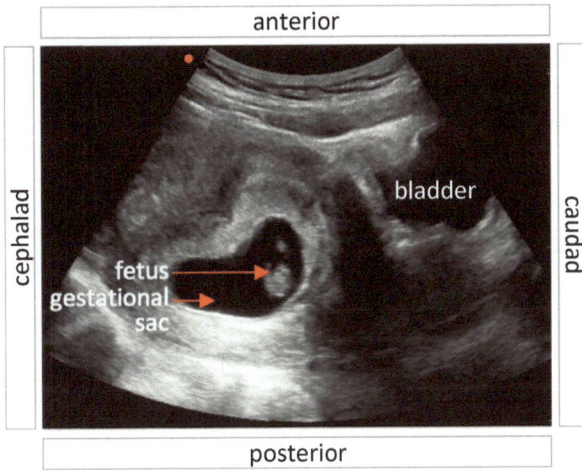

**Video 11.1 Intra-uterine fetal cardiac activity on trans-abdominal ultrasound.**
Video: bedsideultrasoundlevel1.com

### Clinical relevance - Ectopic pregnancy

Ultrasound findings are used in combination with laboratory and clinical assessments in the management of suspected ectopic pregnancy.

In a pregnant patient suspected of having an ectopic pregnancy [51, 53, 54]:

- The presence of an intra-uterine pregnancy excludes an ectopic pregnancy in the vast majority of cases. The exception to this rule is the heterotopic pregnancy (1:4000-8000 normal pregnancies; 1:100 pregnancies with assisted-reproductive techniques) where both intra-uterine and extra-uterine pregnancies occur simultaneously

- The absence of an intra-uterine pregnancy suggests an ectopic pregnancy, particularly after 6 weeks of gestational age

- Unstable vital signs, the absence of an intra-uterine pregnancy, and the presence of free pelvic or intraabdominal fluid (Chapter 6) is compelling evidence for a ruptured ectopic pregnancy.

### Clinical relevance - Other pathology

- **Blighted ovum:** Patients with a blighted ovum will have a positive BHCG without the development of a fetus. The presence of an empty gestational sac with a diameter greater than 25 mm is highly suggestive of a blighted ovum. Pseudogestational sacs are much smaller than 25 mm

- **Molar pregnancy:** Patients with a molar pregnancy often present with the clinical triad of anemia, hyperthyroidism, and hyperemesis. The BHCG is very high. On bedside ultrasound the uterus is full of a multitude of small cystic structures.

## 11.4  Troubleshooting tips

- To improve the quality of pelvic ultrasound images:

    o  Ensure that the patient's bladder is full

    o  Scan in both sagittal and transverse planes

    o  Use the zoom function on your ultrasound machine to better visualize within the gestational sac

- The uterus is usually imaged at a depth of 10-15 cm

- When the uterus is not at the midline, its position is best determined by scanning in the transverse plane

- If the gestational age is later than expected, the pregnant uterus may have entered the abdominal cavity

- If there is any doubt about the presence of an IUP with trans-abdominal scanning, convert to trans-vaginal scanning.

## 11.5   False-positives and false-negatives

Beware false-positives! Declaring an IUP when none exists is a false-positive. Declaring a false-positive IUP when the pregnancy is ectopic is a dangerous error. Ectopic pregnancies are potentially life threatening!

**False-positives (for IUP):**

- **Lacking criteria:** Any case in which not all of the five criteria for diagnosing an intra-uterine pregnancy are present

- **Pseudogestational sac:** A pseudogestational sac in an ectopic pregnancy could be mistaken for an intra-uterine gestational sac

- **Visible ectopic pregnancy:** A visible ectopic pregnancy could be mistaken for an intra-uterine pregnancy. To avoid this error, ensure that all five criteria of IUP are identified.

## 11.6   CPoCUS documentation standards

The Canadian Point of Care Ultrasound Society (CPoCUS) recommends that POCUS exams be documented as follows:

- **First trimester pregnancy:**

  o   Not all criteria for an IUP: POCUS  NDIUP

  o   All criteria for an IUP:       POCUS  IUP

  o   All criteria for an IUP plus FHR>100 BPM:

  POCUS  LIUP


*IUP=*       *Intra-uterine pregnancy*
*NDIUP=*   *No definitive intra-uterine pregnancy*
*LIUP=*     *Live intra-uterine pregnancy*

**Case closed:**

The 30 year old pregnant woman has no intra-uterine pregnancy identified on ultrasound examination. An ectopic pregnancy is suspected. She is transferred for urgent obstetrics consultation.

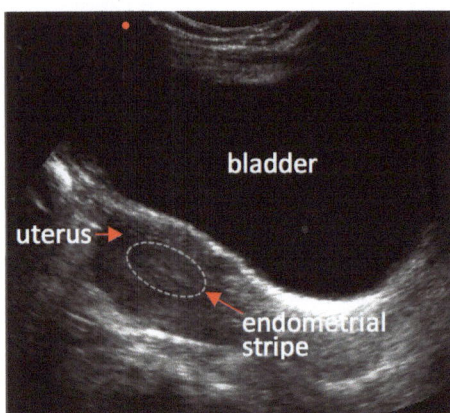

**Figure 11.8 A normal uterus imaged in the sagittal plane.**

# INDEX

## A

A lines · 37, 50, 55
A profile · 52
AAA · 78, 104, 105, 110, 111
AB profile · 52
Abdominal aorta · 105, 106, 107, 108, 109
Abdominal aortic aneurysm · 104, 105, 110, 111
Abdominal setting · 26
Acoustic enhancement · 132
Acute respiratory distress syndrome · 51, 70
Anechoic · 5
Aortic diameter · 112
Artifacts · 31, 32, 33
Ascites · 132
Asthma · 47, 52
Atelectasis · 47
Attenuation · 4, 5, 7, 34

## B

B lines · 51
B profile · 52
BART · 12
Bear paw sign · 146
Bladder · 91, 139, 143, 144, 145, 147, 148, 174, 175
Body planes · 22
Bowel gas · 130

## C

Cardiac lung point · 49
Cardiac setting · 27
Cardiac tamponade · 72
Cholecystitis · 117, 119, 126, 132, 133
Cholelithiasis · 127
Chronic obstructive pulmonary disease · 52, 70
Cirrhosis · 132

Comet tail artifacts · 49
Common femoral artery · 161
Common femoral vein · 156, 158, 159, 160, 161, 162
Compression ultrasound · 156, 158, 164, 165
Congestive heart failure · 132
COPD · 52
Curtain sign · 54
Curvilinear probe · 16

# D

Deep venous thrombosis · 156
Density · 6, 32
Depth · 8, 9, 15, 28, 105, 119, 139, 173
Doppler · 12
DVT · 18, 52, 55, 156, 158, 159, 163, 165
Dyspnea · 37, 41, 42, 43, 52, 53, 55

# E

E lines · 49
Ectopic pregnancy · 78, 171, 172, 173, 180
Edge artifact · 127, 130
eFAST algorithm · 86
Endometrial stripe · 174, 175
Enhancement artifact · 34
Epigastric · 106, 120
Exclamation point sign · 123
Eye · 16

# F

Far-field · 25, 127, 132
Fetal pole · 176, 178
Field of view · 24
Foley catheter · 148
Fractional shortening · 66
Frequency · 1, 4, 10, 11, 12, 15, 16, 24, 43, 63, 85, 105, 119, 139, 157, 173

# G

Gain · 7, 29
Gallbladder · 32, 118, 119, 120, 121, 122, 123, 124, 125, 126, 127, 128, 129, 131, 132, 133
Gallstones · 32, 118, 126, 127
Gel · 19
Gestational sac · 176
Great saphenous vein · 161

# H

Hemopericardium · 86, 95
Hemoperitoneum · 86, 87, 98, 99
Hemothorax · 86, 96
Hepatitis · 132
Heterotopic pregnancy · 180
Hydronephrosis · 145, 146, 148
Hyperdynamic LV function · 69
Hyperechoic · 5
Hypoechoic · 5
Hypoproteinemia · 132

Hypotension · 61, 63, 70, 77, 78

Hypovolemia · 62, 69, 73, 76, 77

## I

Inferior vena cava (IVC) · 8, 26, 73, 74, 75, 107, 108

Interstitial fibrosis · 51

Intraabdominal · 78, 87

Intra-uterine pregnancy · 171, 176, 180

## K

Kidney · 16, 18, 139

Kidney injury · 138

## L

Left lateral decubitus · 120, 121

Left ventricular (LV) function · 69

Left ventricular (LV) dysfunction · 55, 62

Linear probe · 16

Liver · 16

Liver lung point · 49

Lung consolidation · 54

Lung point · 47, 48

Lung sliding · 45, 46, 47, 48, 52, 78

## M

Mid-clavicular line · 44, 120

Mirror image artifact · 36

Morison's pouch · 87, 88, 122

Myocardial infarction · 69, 76, 77

## N

Near-field · 25, 132

## O

Obstructive airways disease · 50

Orientation marker · 26

## P

Patient position · 15, 17, 18

Pelvic fluid · 87, 91

Pelvis · 87, 91, 92, 93

Penetration · 10, 11

Pericardial effusion · 61, 71

Phased array probe · 16

Pleural adhesions · 47

Pleural effusion · 5, 54, 55, 56, 86, 96

Pneumonia · 51, 52, 55

Pneumothorax · 45, 46, 47, 78, 86, 97

Popliteal vein · 164, 165

Posterolateral approach · 120, 122

Postprandial state · 132

Post-renal failure · 138
Post-void bladder volume · 147
Pouch of Douglas · 91, 93
Probe · 3
Pulmonary edema · 51, 52
Pulmonary embolism · 52, 62,
    70, 76, 77

## R

Reflection · 5
Refraction (edge) artifact · 38,
    127, 130
Renal failure · 132
Resolution · 1, 10, 11
Respiratory variability · 75
Reverberation artifact · 37
Rib shadows · 44, 51, 152
Ruling in pneumothorax · 47
Ruling out pneumothorax · 45
Ruptured ectopic pregnancy ·
    180
RV-LV ratio · 77, 78

## S

Sepsis · 77
Shadow · 32, 33, 107, 127, 128
Shadowing artifact · 32
Sonographic Murphy sign · 131
Spine sign · 55, 96
Spleen · 16
Spleno-renal space · 87, 89, 90
Subcostal sweep · 120
Symphysis pubis · 91, 92, 143,
    144, 174, 175

## T

Tachycardia · 69
Tamponade · 62, 72, 76, 77
Testicle · 16
Tibioperoneal trunk · 164
Trans-abdominal pelvic
    ultrasound · 172
Transvaginal ultrasound · 173
Trauma · 78, 83, 84, 85, 86, 94,
    95, 96, 97

## U

Ultrasound · 1
Undifferentiated hypotension ·
    62, 63
Unilateral bronchial intubation ·
    47
Uterus · 91, 174, 175, 176, 178

## V

Vertebral body · 6, 8, 26, 107,
    108

## W

WES sign · 127, 129

## X

X-7 approach · 120, 121

## Y

Yolk sac · 176, 178

# REFERENCES

1.    Lanctôt J-F, Valois M and Beaulieu Y. EGLS: Echo-guided life support. An algorithmic approach to undifferentiated shock. *Crit Ultrasound J.* 2011; 3:123-129.

2.    Mrabet Y. Human_anatomy_planes.svg. *Wikimedia Commons.* 2012.

3.    Lichtenstein DA. Pneumothorax. *Whole body ultrasonography in the critically ill.* Berlin Heidelberg: Springer, 2010, p. 163-179.

4.    Lichtenstein DA and Menu Y. A bedside ultrasound sign ruling out pneumothorax in the critically ill. Lung sliding. *Chest.* 1995; 108:1345-1348.

5.    Kirkpatrick AW, Sirois M, Laupland KB, et al. Hand-held thoracic sonography for detecting post-traumatic pneumothoraces: the Extended Focused Assessment with Sonography for Trauma (EFAST). *J Trauma.* 2004; 57:288-295.

6.    Lichtenstein DA, Meziere G, Lascols N, et al. Ultrasound diagnosis of occult pneumothorax. *Crit Care Med.* 2005; 33:1231-1238.

7.    Noble VE, Nelson B and Sutingco AN. Focused asessment with sonography in Trauma (FAST). *Manual of emergency and critical care ultrasound.* New York: Cambridge University Press, 2007, p. 23-51.

8.   Piette E, Daoust R and Denault A. Basic concepts in the use of thoracic and lung ultrasound. *Curr Opin Anaesthesiol.* 2013; 26:20-30.

9.   Lichtenstein D, Meziere G, Biderman P and Gepner A. The "lung point": an ultrasound sign specific to pneumothorax. *Intensive Care Med.* 2000; 26:1434-1440.

10.  Lichtenstein D. Introduction to lung ultrasound. *Whole body ultrasonography in the critically ill.* Berlin Heidelberg: Springer, 2010, p. 117-127.

11.  Lichtenstein D and Meziere G. A lung ultrasound sign allowing bedside distinction between pulmonary edema and COPD: the comet-tail artifact. *Intensive Care Med.* 1998; 24:1331-1334.

12.  Lichtenstein DA and Meziere GA. Relevance of lung ultrasound in the diagnosis of acute respiratory failure: the BLUE protocol. *Chest.* 2008; 134:117-125.

13.  Yang PC, Luh KT, Chang DB, et al. Value of sonography in determining the nature of pleural effusion: analysis of 320 cases. *AJR Am J Roentgenol.* 1992; 159:29-33.

14.  Anderson B. Two-dimensional echocardiographic measurements and calculations. *Echocardiography: The normal examination and echocardiographic measurements.* Brisbane, Australia2000, p. 87-104.

15.  Amico AF, Lichtenberg GS, Reisner SA, et al. Superiority of visual versus computerized echocardiographic estimation of radionuclide left ventricular ejection fraction. *Am Heart J.* 1989; 118:1259-1265.

16.  Mueller X, Stauffer JC, Jaussi A, Goy JJ and Kappenberger L. Subjective visual echocardiographic estimate of left ventricular ejection fraction as an alternative to conventional echocardiographic methods: comparison with contrast angiography. *Clin Cardiol.* 1991; 14:898-902.

17.  Randazzo MR, Snoey ER, Levitt MA and Binder K. Accuracy of emergency physician assessment of left ventricular ejection

fraction and central venous pressure using echocardiography. *Acad Emerg Med.* 2003; 10:973-977.

18.   Stamm RB, Carabello BA, Mayers DL and Martin RP. Two-dimensional echocardiographic measurement of left ventricular ejection fraction: prospective analysis of what constitutes an adequate determination. *Am Heart J.* 1982; 104:136-144.

19.   Jardin F, Dubourg O and Bourdarias JP. Echocardiographic pattern of acute cor pulmonale. *Chest.* 1997; 111:209-217.

20.   Reardon RF and Joing SA. Cardiac. In: Ma OJ, Mateer JR and Blaivas M, (eds.). *Emergency Ultrasound.* 2nd ed. USA: McGraw Hill, 2008, p. 110-148.

21.   Jackson RE, Rudoni RR, Hauser AM, Pascual RG and Hussey ME. Prospective evaluation of two-dimensional transthoracic echocardiography in emergency department patients with suspected pulmonary embolism. *Acad Emerg Med.* 2000; 7:994-998.

22.   Lyon M, Blaivas M and Brannam L. Sonographic measurement of the inferior vena cava as a marker of blood loss. *Am J Emerg Med.* 2005; 23:45-50.

23.   Natori H, Tamaki S and Kira S. Ultrasonographic evaluation of ventilatory effect on inferior vena caval configuration. *Am Rev Respir Dis.* 1979; 120:421-427.

24.   Simonson JS and Schiller NB. Sonospirometry: a new method for noninvasive estimation of mean right atrial pressure based on two-dimensional echographic measurements of the inferior vena cava during measured inspiration. *J Am Coll Cardiol.* 1988; 11:557-564.

25.   Kircher BJ, Himelman RB and Schiller NB. Noninvasive estimation of right atrial pressure from the inspiratory collapse of the inferior vena cava. *Am J Cardiol.* 1990; 66:493-496.

26.   Ommen SR, Nishimura RA, Hurrell DG and Klarich KW. Assessment of right atrial pressure with 2-dimensional and Doppler echocardiography: a simultaneous catheterization and echocardiographic study. *Mayo Clin Proc.* 2000; 75:24-29.

27.   Wong SP. Echocardiographic findings in acute and chronic pulmonary disease. In: Otto CM, (ed.). *The practice of clinical echocardiography*. 2nd edition ed. Philadelphia: W.B. Saunders Company, 2002, p. 739-760.

28.   Tayal VS and Kendall JL. Trauma. In: Cosby KS and Kendall JL, (eds.). *Practical guide to emergency ultrasound*. Philadelphia: Lippincott Williams & Wilkins, 2006, p. 43-92.

29.   Ma O and Mateer J. Trauma. In: Ma OJ, Mateer JR and Blaivas M, (eds.). *Emergency Ultrasound*. USA: McGraw Hill, 2008, p. 77-108.

30.   Socransky S and Wiss R. *Essential of point-of-care ultrasound "The EDE Book"*. 2015.

31.   Ouellet JF, Ball CG, Panebianco NL and Kirkpatrick AW. The sonographic diagnosis of pneumothorax. *J Emerg Trauma Shock*. 2011; 4:504-507.

32.   Noble VE, Nelson B and Sutingco AN. Abdominal aortic aneurysm. *Manual of emergency and critical care ultrasound*. New York: Cambridge University Press, 2007, p. 105-118.

33.   Reardon RF, Cook T and Plummer D. Abdominal aortic aneurysm. In: Ma OJ, Mateer JR and Blaivas M, (eds.). *Emergency Ultrasound*. USA: McGraw Hill, 2008, p. 149-167.

34.   Tayal VS, Graf CD and Gibbs MA. Prospective study of accuracy and outcome of emergency ultrasound for abdominal aortic aneurysm over two years. *Acad Emerg Med*. 2003; 10:867-871.

35.   Shuman WP, Hastrup W, Jr., Kohler TR, et al. Suspected leaking abdominal aortic aneurysm: use of sonography in the emergency room. *Radiology*. 1988; 168:117-119.

36.   Engel JM, Deitch EA and Sikkema W. Gallbladder wall thickness: sonographic accuracy and relation to disease. *AJR Am J Roentgenol*. 1980; 134:907-909.

37.   Finberg HJ and Birnholz JC. Ultrasound evaluation of the gallbladder wall. *Radiology*. 1979; 133:693-698.

38.    Bree RL. Further observations on the usefulness of the sonographic Murphy sign in the evaluation of suspected acute cholecystitis. *J Clin Ultrasound*. 1995; 23:169-172.

39.    Ralls PW, Halls J, Lapin SA, et al. Prospective evaluation of the sonographic Murphy sign in suspected acute cholecystitis. *J Clin Ultrasound*. 1982; 10:113-115.

40.    Ralls PW, Colletti PM, Lapin SA, et al. Real-time sonography in suspected acute cholecystitis. Prospective evaluation of primary and secondary signs. *Radiology*. 1985; 155:767-771.

41.    Swadron S and Mandavia D. Renal. In: Ma OJ, Mateer JR and Blaivas M, (eds.). *Emergency Ultrasound*. USA: McGraw Hill, 2008, p. 230-255.

42.    Byrne M, Kimberly H and Noble VE. Emergency renal ultrasonography. In: Adams JG, Barton ED, Collings J, DeBlieux PMC, Gisondi MA and MNadel ES, (eds.). *Emergency medicine: Clinical essentials*. Saunders, 2013, p. 998-1002.

43.    Kelly CE. Evaluation of voiding dysfunction and measurement of bladder volume. *Rev Urol*. 2004; 6 Suppl 1:S32-37.

44.    Chan H. Noninvasive bladder volume measurement. *J Neurosci Nurs*. 1993; 25:309-312.

45.    Birdwell BG, Raskob GE, Whitsett TL, et al. The clinical validity of normal compression ultrasonography in outpatients suspected of having deep venous thrombosis. *Ann Intern Med*. 1998; 128:1-7.

46.    Blaivas M, Lambert MJ, Harwood RA, Wood JP and Konicki J. Lower-extremity Doppler for deep venous thrombosis--can emergency physicians be accurate and fast? *Acad Emerg Med*. 2000; 7:120-126.

47.    Magazzini S, Vanni S, Toccafondi S, et al. Duplex ultrasound in the emergency department for the diagnostic management of clinically suspected deep vein thrombosis. *Acad Emerg Med*. 2007; 14:216-220.

48.    Poppiti R, Papanicolaou G, Perese S and Weaver FA. Limited B-mode venous imaging versus complete color-flow duplex venous

scanning for detection of proximal deep venous thrombosis. *J Vasc Surg*. 1995; 22:553-557.

49.    Theodoro D, Blaivas M, Duggal S, Snyder G and Lucas M. Real-time B-mode ultrasound in the ED saves time in the diagnosis of deep vein thrombosis (DVT). *Am J Emerg Med*. 2004; 22:197-200.

50.    Labropoulos N and Tassiopoulos AK. Vascular diagnosis of venous thrombosis. In: Mansour MA and Labropoulos N, (eds.). *Vascular diagnosis*. Philadelphia: Elsevier Saunders, 2005, p. 429-438.

51.    Middleton WD, Kurtz AB and Hertzberg BS. The first trimester and ectopic pregnancy. *Ultrasound: The Requisites*. St-Louis, MI: Mosby, 2004, p. 342-373.

52.    Noble VE, Nelson B and Sutingco AN. First trimester ultrasound. *Manual of emergency and critical care ultrasound*. New York: Cambridge University Press, 2007, p. 85-103.

53.    Nordenholz K, Abbott J and Bailitz J. First trimester pregnancy. In: Cosby KS and Kendall JL, (eds.). *Practical guide to emergency ultrasound*. Philadelphia: Lippincott Williams & Wilkins, 2006, p. 124-160.

54.    Reardon RF and Joing SA. Frist trimester pregnancy. In: Ma OJ, Mateer JR and Blaivas M, (eds.). *Emergency Ultrasound*. USA: McGraw Hill, 2008, p. 179-318.